Monica Jay w[as born in Poland and has] lived in Lond[on for m]ost of her life. She immersed herself in the study of problems of early childhood development when one of her own children turned out to be a borderline autistic, and she subsequently ran her own Montessori nursery school. She is registered with the Birmingham Social Services as a counsellor for transvestites and their families nationwide, and she also counsels for the Beaumont Trust and the Transvestite/ Transsexual Social Group of London.

Geraldine

The Story of a Transvestite

MONICA JAY

Mandarin

A Mandarin Paperback
GERALDINE

First published in Great Britain 1985
by Caliban Books
This revised edition published 1992
by Mandarin Paperbacks
Michelin House, 81 Fulham Road, London SW3 6RB

Mandarin is an imprint of Reed Consumer Books Ltd

Copyright © Monica Jay 1985, 1992

A CIP catalogue record for this title
is available from the British Library
ISBN 0 7493 3604 8

Printed and bound in Great Britain
by Cox & Wyman Ltd, Reading, Berks.

This book is sold subject to the condition
that it shall not, by way of trade or otherwise,
be lent, resold, hired out, or otherwise circulated
without the publisher's prior consent in any form
of binding or cover other than that in which
it is published and without a similar condition
including this condition being imposed
on the subsequent purchaser.

In writing the story of my love for a transvestite I do not presume to have all the answers to the enigma of transvestism. No complete understanding of this subject can exist while the majority of men who have this compulsion are hiding it and rarely if ever 'come out', but the chances are that there are one or two living down your road. The transvestite is not the odd man out. A transvestite could be your best friend, your butcher, your solicitor, your boss, your husband, your son, your brother – or your lover.

Transvestism:
**A tendency to dress
in the clothes of the
opposite sex.**
Penguin English Dictionary

I

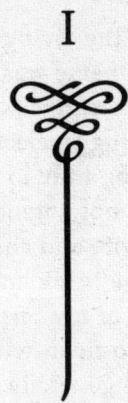

It was a shivery February afternoon in 1982 and I was in the middle of tidying up my front room when the doorbell rang. The latest applicant in search of a bedsit had arrived on my doorstep.

Apprehensive, I hurried to let him in, shutting the door again quickly to keep out the cold. I beckoned him inside to a seat in the warm room, giving myself time to assess him: he was youngish, probably in his early thirties, lively, intelligent, well-spoken, cheerful. His black winter coat was well-cut. So far, so good. It was the eyes alone which gave me a feeling of unease: set deep in his handsome face with the swarthy dark looks of a buccaneer they were jet-black and extraordinarily intense, cutting through my landladyish defences and putting me off my guard.

He followed me upstairs to inspect the tiny room.

Yes, he liked it. It contained a spacious wardrobe, a comfortable bed and, hanging from the wall, a large removable mirror.

Back downstairs in the living room the interview went in his favour. His name was Gerald Tilson and he was starting out in an executive position with a London business firm specialising in electronics. Home was in the country, too far for him to commute. Plausible. But why then did he not intend to go back for the weekends to be with wife and children? I guessed that the marriage was on the brink and that he was here to sort himself out. None of my business. All I was looking for was someone to fit in with the rest of us, pay the rent promptly, and generally behave in a civilised way, and this man looked as if he might fit the bill. My short experience as a landlady had already shown me that such a person was none too easy to come by – solitary women are vulnerable to predators, and some of my paying guests had turned out to be simply ghastly.

He moved in on the following Saturday and at once began to liven up the scene in the dining room, where we all congregated in the mornings over cornflakes and toast.

He started to come down after the rest of us had assembled, all charm and easy smiles, making straight for the large mirror facing the dining table while still knotting his tie, introducing into our little circle a feeling of cosy intimacy. No sooner had he joined us than he would have us in fits with his risqué jokes, sparked off by the presence of two women. Gerald, we were unanimous, was an absolute darling, even if he did have sex on the brain, and the room was strangely lifeless until he made his appearance.

Supervising my little group from the direction of the cooker and making sure that everyone left for work well fed, my arms folded over my red PVC apron, I felt pleased. Now, for the first time since my divorce and in my new role as a landlady, I had got an admirable team together: Dorothy, middle-aged, amiable and mild-mannered and sharing her room with a crazy cat, was in the process of freeing herself from an unsatisfactory husband. Dave, the solid civil servant from Birmingham was slowly finding his feet in London, and now there was Gerald to add spice to the mixture.

He lost no time at all in making himself thoroughly at home by starting to use my fridge at any time he fancied, and soon afterwards by declaring that he was not prepared to forego his favourite programme, *Minder*. Not having much liking for crooks myself, I withdrew ostentatiously each time, making my silent protest, but he could not have cared less. Glued to the box and doubling up with laughter whenever one of his heroes made a scoop, he had a lovely time sitting in my favourite seat, seemingly without a care in the world.

Still, he made up for it. He much admired and praised the way I had converted the appalling wreck of a house I had purchased, a sure and straight way to my heart. He complimented me on the way I had planned and arranged it all, with myself snugly dug into my warm and colourful home downstairs, while upstairs my paying guests made sure that I could keep my head above water. Gerald, after all, was a darling.

Slowly things were falling into place for me.

'We have a lot to talk about,' Gerald had assured me soon after he had moved in, on discovering that I had a continental background and spoke German and French, two languages which he himself had mastered fluently, having worked abroad for some years. 'Oh yes?' I had thought. My newly won freedom from married slavery and my soaring confidence as an independent woman had made me very suspicious of men. I found that I could get on a lot better without them. In my fairly new role as a landlady I had certainly learned to be very cautious: I was a woman and alone, and therefore exposed to cranks, paranoids, and generally to people who liked to shift their problems on to me.

But Gerald appealed to me instantly when talking about his two young children, Emily and Tommy. His eyes lit up the moment he mentioned them, loving to describe them in all their minutest ways. Emily at six, long-legged and endowed with her father's dark hair and eyes, was a most pretty little girl, and already quite a help in the home, eager to give her mother a hand by laying the table and helping Daddy to clear it all up afterwards. Tommy was a very sturdy little fellow who took after his mother with his blonde curls and her wide blue eyes. At four he was a most determined little chap who knew how to stand his ground firmly. Soon I could picture them both vividly, enabling me to get a glimpse of the domestic scene Gerald had left behind. He had taken Emily to school each morning on his way to work, looking forward to reading stories to them both on his return at night. And weekends were filled with games, kicking balls, romping about in the fields.

'No one seeing those children could help loving them,' he said. I found myself envying those two their wonderful warm Daddy, the kind of Daddy which my own children had never known.

Emily had saved up her pocket money for weeks to give her Daddy a birthday present. She had planned it all on her own. When the moment came her face and eyes had lit up and she had been quite out of breath when handing him the packet, unable to contain for another moment her impatience to see his joy. The hugs, the laughter, the kisses. 'Happy birthday, Daddy,' Emily and Tommy had sung, and Gerald was never to forget the scene.

Upstairs by his bedside stood the two cards: Emily's colourful drawing and laborious signature, and Tommy's cheerful scribble. They were never removed.

He had been right, we did have a lot to talk about. Gerald in his more serious moods revealed a surprising sense of perception. Behind his cheerful veneer he was lonely, he missed the children and he missed Erika, his lovely wife. In the corner of his bedsit, on top of the bookshelf, stood a large picture of her: cool, blonde and attractive, she made her presence felt. Gerald was disorientated, and he hated his new job.

Trying to combat his loneliness he started to come

down to me in the empty evenings, gin-and-tonic in hand, cigarette dangling, offering his endearing company to me and intruding on the isolation which for the past four years I had guarded with such dogged determination while licking my bruises and shaping my new life.

What incomparable fun Gerald turned out to be, though! Filling the room to the brim with his person, his charisma almost knocking me off my feet, wit and sparkle abounding, he lost no time whatever in chasing my loneliness out of the window with a vengeance.

He was so widely travelled, his German and French so perfect, including a fair knowledge of Swiss and Italian, he struck me more as a Middle European than the prototype of an expensively educated Englishman; certainly there seemed nothing very conventional about him. His mind was so flexible, he could turn it to anything he liked with the greatest of ease and talk about it in depth. In the past I had rarely if ever had the pleasure of being in the company of such an adaptable mind.

Soon he started to make himself useful to me: a man who would happily get on with even the most complicated tasks round the house was something quite new to me. Gerald turned out to be a superman. One Sunday, returning from a country visit in tatty slacks and ancient jumper, I found him still there, tiling my newly erected bathroom. In my immense gratitude I reached up to him, offering him a peck on the cheek and he responded eagerly like a hungry puppy starved of affection, but I left it at that. He was just not for me, much too young, much too gorgeous, too charming, too everything, and anyway, I was his landlady and I knew my place. But I promised to cook him a meal some day.

And he was full of surprises. One day as we walked up the High Street together he suddenly turned round: 'Do you wear a corset?' he wanted to know. I looked at him, highly amused. 'Are you crazy?' I laughed. 'Listen, my own mother threw hers into the fire when she was seventeen, and anyway, we are now living in the twentieth century!'

He did not pursue this particular theme, though he began to give me little face creams, hand creams, moisture masks. Great fun – no man had ever indulged me like this before, and although they were only samples, I still felt thrilled with them. Dear Gerald, I could certainly go along with that! And before I had time to reflect, I found myself sitting in the beauty salon of our local fashion store, purring under a make-up session, my first ever.

Re-emerging after an hour's intensive attention to my eyes, lips, cheekbones and neck, my colouring much enhanced and certainly attracting the attention of quite a few passers-by, I suddenly bumped into my good old friend Louisa. Louisa knew about my weak spot for Gerald, understood, and in no time at all we were both convulsed with hysterics. If the make-up session had perhaps not done much else for me, those shrieks of laughter alone were well worth all the trouble.

Louisa took me home to lunch in her sophisticated flat overlooking the riverside at Richmond where she lived with her husband James and their teenage daughter. We had our bread and cheese in her kitchen, spreading ourselves over the large wooden table, Louisa supplying me with plenty of white wine, my favourite. No shortage in her house, James being in the wine business. I did not have many secrets from Louisa, although she is much more conventional than me, but not stodgily so, and mellowed by a keen sense of humour. Pouring me glass after glass of the white wine she soon had me in a wonderfully relaxed and romantic mood and talking about Gerald, whom she had not yet met. In vain I searched for words to describe adequately to her this breathtaking phenomenon who was my latest paying guest. 'I just know that if I were to travel to the end of the globe I could not possibly, ever, meet a man who excited me more,' I said finally, this being the best I could do. Louisa burst into peals of laughter: 'You have a 31-year-old on the brain,' she said.

It suddenly brought it home to me – she was right, I had! Sobering up later, I thought how silly I had been.

'You have a lot to give,' said Gerald to me one night while we were facing one another over drinks in the living room as usual, smiling his most charming smile, and there was a warmth and a caress in his voice which alerted me. It was true, I had a great deal of life experience – the question was, who to give it to?

By now I had begun to look forward eagerly to my evenings with Gerald. Our conversation flowed so effortlessly, and it was thrilling to have this beautiful charismatic man all to myself.

He was barely older than my own eldest son and

came from a background of public school and strict parents living in the grand manner, whereas I had had a continental upbringing by affectionate but poor artist parents, with a disrupted education and flight from the Nazi madness; but this made no difference at all to the fact that we viewed the world as one. We were strong individuals both, sensitive to a fault and vulnerable, both of us trying to present a tough and brave face to the outside world; we were both ambitious in our own ways, determined to persevere in the face of great obstacles; we were both strugglers, we both craved for a big challenge. We bridged that age gap with ease.

'You are a very attractive lady!' Gerald said to me another night. Me? True, I did not look my age, nor feel it. I was strong, resilient, and had perfect health. And of course, I felt flattered.

I took my first ever picture of Gerald around this time – he had come down one day on the way to an old boys' reunion and suddenly there he stood, dark dinner jacket, bow-tie, dark eyes and hair, dazzling against the whitewashed wall. WOW! I rushed to grab my camera, to immortalise this breathtaking vision, standing there smiling so self-consciously, showing himself to me – showing himself *off* to me?

A couple of days later I was busily pottering about in the kitchen. The day was warm and sunny, there was a soothing breeze in the air, and the birds were chirping in the garden with all their might. Suddenly there floated through the open window the unearthly sounds of James Galway playing his Magic Flute. I hurried to open the front door to find out the source of these extraordinary sounds, and saw Gerald. There he sat in his car, one arm dangling out of the window, his beautiful face relaxed, listening to his latest tape, and I could just make out an open bottle of wine on the seat next to him. No one had ever before managed to transport our very ordinary road with its terraced houses and parked cars into a site of such happiness; it was as if someone had poured a bucket of gold over it all, making every stone sing.

I think that this is the moment when I first fell in love with him.

Love for a man – how it had always frightened me! Ever since that day so long ago when I had come across it for the very first time. It had happened in Berlin, in the early thirties. I was holding on to my mother's hand, a little girl of seven or eight, dressed in the dark brown velvet coat she had made for me, with sheepskin trimmings and a little hat to match. I must have looked very pretty with my large dark eyes and masses of curls and I skipped along merrily in the sunny street, when towards us walked a tall, slim and handsome man, elegantly clothed in a long fawn coat, a trilby on his head. As he came nearer he smiled at me long and tenderly, in all likelihood remembering his own little girl back home. The little Eve inside me, waiting, had been stirred but I never saw him again, and because of it I discovered at a very tender age the futility of love. Love for a man meant hurt, disappointment, and therefore it was dangerous and best avoided.

Up till now I had managed, more or less successfully, to run away from the perils of a great passion, scared of my own feelings.

Then, one night, reclining on the sofa with a gin-and-tonic before him as always, and me squatting on the ground at his feet, Gerald announced that he wanted to make a 'confession', overriding all my objections. I do not like confessions. People are carried away by the temptation of the moment to get things off their chest, only to feel embarrassed the following day. I did not want Gerald to be embarrassed with me. I did not want him to move out of my house.

But there was no stopping him. He came straight to the point. 'You said you have had lots of odd people going through your house,' he said. 'I bet you have never had a transvestite.'

'No,' I said.

'I am a transvestite,' said Gerald.

There flashed through my mind the fragments of a play I had once watched on the television, of a handsome tall youth in long blonde wig and female dress, visiting a club where he met with others like himself and falling in love with the girl attendant, and they lived happily ever after.

'You're having me on, Gerald, you're joking!' I tried in vain to stem the laughter that was welling up inside me. 'Why on earth should a gorgeous-looking man like yourself want to turn himself into a woman?' I didn't believe a word of it. This extraordinary and certainly very manly Gerald with his superb sense of humour had just found a new way to make me laugh.

But Gerald looked at me, smiling, his expressive dark eyes serious. I studied this fascinating face before me for give-away signs of teasing. I found none. He was serious! How very strange, how extraordinary! Gerald in woman's dress? It made no sense at all.

When Gerald further confessed to having gone out the previous night to a club dressed as a woman, describing himself in all the details, an overwhelming desire to giggle came over me at the thought of him stealing down my respectable staircase dressed like this, in wig, dress, handbag, high heels, make-up, the lot, at dead of night. My giggles gathered momentum and turned into a crazed hysterical avalanche of laughter which I could no longer control, the picture before my eyes incredible, hilarious.

Gerald, however, did not flinch. 'I suppose this is the best thing to do,' he shrugged his shoulders in some resignation, 'have a good laugh at it.' Little did I know then of the shame and deep despair which my laughter was causing him.

It seemed a very long time indeed before I was able to regain my senses and curb that laughter. At long last I began to calm down. And now I tried to come to grips with Gerald's dilemma. As he was so inordinately fond of women, I suggested, perhaps dressing himself as one was an attempt on his part to feel himself into the role of the opposite sex, to come closer to understanding women? Gerald, however, did not take to the idea. No, this was not what made him a transvestite.

Another thought now formed itself in my mind. Did he, perhaps, possess some female hormones which prompted him to act as a woman from time to time? Gerald had absolutely no hesitation on this one: *'No!'* he said, firmly, and that was that.

The fact that I 'knew' did not affect my attitude towards Gerald. He had a quirk – so what? This made him no less the person whom I liked enormously and for whom – alas – I found myself developing feelings which in the light of our immense age gap began to disturb me. Our intimate talks until the early hours of the morning accompanied by drinks and music had become the most exciting events in my solitary existence. I decided it was best to avoid him, however painful that might turn out to be.

Putting my decision into practice with a heavy heart, two dreary weeks dragged by. In the mornings we met over breakfast as usual, always in the company of Dorothy and Dave, with myself strictly in my role as a landlady, but in the evenings I roamed the neighbourhood, surprising friends and relatives alike, frequenting the local cinema, not daring to make my way back home until all danger of meeting Gerald had safely passed.

Still, how long can you avoid your own home? Apart from everything else I longed for my creature comforts, missed eating my evening meal in my own dining room, missed seeing my favourite programme on the box, missed hearing the phone ring.

But on my very first night back home, there he stood in the doorway smiling, eyes and mouth beguiling, rendering me defenceless within seconds. 'I have missed you, Mona!' he greeted me. 'Where have you been?' I thought that I was hearing the purest of pure music.

'Would you care for a drink and a chat?' he offered eagerly. And indeed there was nothing, just nothing under the sun I would have liked better, and so I settled myself on the floor as usual and waited for Gerald to reappear. He came down, gin-and-tonic in hand, and sat by me, looking more darkly enticing than ever.

I suppose it was after all inevitable that Gerald should steer the conversation ever closer towards the topics of love and sex, while I, trying my hardest to keep remote, smiled at him my most maternal smile: the urges and preoccupations of an excitable young man, nothing whatever to do with me!

Useless! Gerald's charisma and compelling magnetism rendered me weak and helpless. I felt the ground giving under me. With an overwhelming feeling of relief and abandonment I finally allowed myself the wonderful luxury of succumbing to his verbal lovemaking, letting it enter every pore of mine, surrendering to the warm sensual pleasure of it.

Even so it came like a complete bolt from the blue

when Gerald, the hour well past midnight, looked down at me sitting at his feet and declared, 'Mona, I want to go to bed with you!' I spun round, amazed, and almost shouted at him, unable to believe what I had just heard: 'Do you realise I could be your mother?' I thought I saw him flinch for a moment, but no, he just turned to smile at me, his boyish face reassuring: 'It makes no difference, Mona, no difference at all!' was all he said.

And so it came about that in spite of our vastly different backgrounds and an age gap spanning a generation, Gerald followed me to my bedroom containing the virginal single pine bed which was my pride, having at long last rid myself of the double bed of evil memories.

But the memories inside me were by no means extinct. A traumatic marriage takes its toll, and mine had crippled me. I had led a solitary and celibate existence for well over a decade, had suffered humiliations and degradation in plenty and now, finding myself face to face with Gerald in the intimacy of my bedroom, prayed that here might be my chance to love, to give, to worship and adore, and perhaps to become a whole woman again. Quite unbeknown to either of us, we were about to take our first step towards what was to become a year of extraordinary and overwhelming experiences for us both.

Neither of us had the slightest inkling of what lay ahead. Gerald, in spite of his *laissez-faire* airs and contagious humour was a deeply shaken man, desperately worried about losing his family – how could we possibly foresee the consequences of our emotional and physical merging?

As it happened, our first fumbling embraces, embarked upon with such high hopes, ended in a succession of mutual shocks, our bed a battlefield, no bed of roses! Where was that romantic lover I had imagined Gerald to be? Casting my mind back over an eternity of years to the loves I had enjoyed then, he did not fit into any pattern I knew. Certainly no man had ever expected me to issue him with an order for sex! In vain I tried to steer Gerald towards a more loving approach, but he was adamant: no order, no sex!

It made me feel puzzled and humiliated. Yet I was aching to love this man and therefore, hesitantly and utterly ashamed of myself, I gave him his orders, freeing him of all responsibility, and with a sigh of relief, whispering endearments in passing, he emerged the winner.

Though not triumphant! Standing over me afterwards, looking down at me, Gerald appeared deep in thought. My own admiration for his physical perfection, however, knew no bounds: no Michelangelo, no Rodin could have found a model more worthy of their immortal works of art. Beautiful from the top of his head down to his toes, his strong broad shoulders tapering off to a slim and boyish waist, to firm and slender thighs, he glowed all over with a rich and golden sheen.

'You must be the most gorgeous man that ever was!' I whispered softly, utterly lost in admiration. To my surprise Gerald's eyes narrowed angrily: 'NO,' he practically hissed at me as if to parry an insult. 'No, I am NOT a gorgeous man!' Taken aback, but full of the courage of my conviction, I insisted nevertheless, 'Oh yes,' I assured him, 'Oh, but I think you are!' And so, long before I could realise what role I would eventually have to play in Gerald's life, I had unknowingly taken my first step towards healing him.

Our first confused trial at lovemaking over, it was now Gerald's turn to avoid me. The next evening was Dorothy's farewell party before moving on, just the four of us at the local pub. Gerald's embarrassment was evident. He, usually the life and soul of any party, was as quiet as a dormouse, barely glancing in my direction all night. On our return home he made a quick dash upstairs, leaving me bewildered and lonely and wondering if by 'giving in' I had now lost a wonderful friend.

A succession of frustrating and agonising days went by, until one day he asked to talk to me to clear the air. After all, we were still living under the same roof and I served up his breakfast as usual every morning. For me it was painful to watch him from a distance, sensing his confusion.

He came to meet me in the living room for the confrontation and worded matters carefully. 'You,' he said, 'see things through older, wiser eyes,' which was true after all, and fair enough. But when he began shifting the blame for the seduction over to me, my blood rose very swiftly. Indeed! Not so very long ago, when leaving my brutally insensitive husband, I had vowed: no mere male was going to mess *me* about again, ever! I had taken all the hurt I was going to take and that was that. I decided to put Gerald in his place there and then.

I looked at him, 'Let's get one thing quite clear,' I said, my voice icy, 'it was not *I* who staged the seduction scene!' Inside I was seething with anger.

To my great surprise he succumbed at once, his eyes softening. Altogether I thought his response odd. It was not until much later that I learned of his craving for the Dominant Woman and the enjoyment he derived from being subdued by her. The fact that I was his landlady had already been a point in favour for me; now I was also proving myself to be forceful and strong.

Nevertheless, Gerald's conscience continued to nag him; he felt he had taken advantage of me, he was ill at ease with himself, and in spite of everything he still felt guilty towards his wife, and so we arrived at a mutual agreement: we decided not to be lovers.

Lying in bed at night, my ears atuned to his movements, I once heard Gerald return home in the early hours of the morning. He had gone and tried his luck with some woman – she had pursued him ever since he had stumbled across her during his house-hunting expedition – he left without a wish ever to see her again. Sex with an attractive woman was great and it was fun, but it was not enough. With a nature such as his Gerald needed more than a mere body to satisfy him.

How could I know at this stage that in his loneliness upstairs Gerald was enacting almost nightly the bizarre and frustrating ritual of the closet transvestite?

II

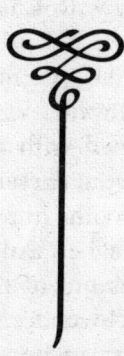

Gerald had started to cross-dress one day when he was fourteen. He had wandered into his mother's bedroom, opened a drawer, taken out some of her underwear and put it on himself. He had lain himself down on his bed feeling marvellously relaxed in the soft garments and without a warning had suddenly had an orgasm, his first ever, and from that day on had dreamed about repeating the experience.

He was brought up by a stern and conventional father, strict and quite incapable of showing warmth, and a kind but unemotional and equally conventional mother. His parents sent him to board in one of the big public schools where he did not particularly excel, in the way that very clever people often do not, but loved games and was popular with the other boys.

He liked to have fun with girls from an early age,

and there were plenty of willing partners around. He also enjoyed walking in the country with his dog and a gun, being at one with himself and his environment, letting his imagination roam. When still in his early twenties he fell in love with Erika, a beautiful blonde, and they married. Gerald believed that his transvestite compulsion would vanish with married life, and indeed for a while all seemed well, but after some months of respite the urge returned with a vengeance. He dealt with it by dreaming about dressing in female clothing, and the dream would soothe him and send him to sleep at night. Occasionally, when Erika was away he would get his bits and pieces out of their hiding place and dress *en femme* and feel wonderful.

The bubble was sure to burst one day. Erika and the children had gone away and Gerald had taken advantage of their absence by cross-dressing and, using the family washing machine for some of his female underwear, had left a pair of frilly knickers behind. When Erika discovered them in the machine she was outraged. A terrible and heartbreaking scene was the result, and Erika accused Gerald of deceiving her with another woman.

Had Gerald perhaps subconsciously manoeuvred the situation so as to have to face up to Erika and come clean? The burden of carrying his lonely secret must have been crushing. He did not know of any other transvestites, and felt all alone with his guilt and his shame and the terror of being ridiculed.

He was now forced to come out into the open and tell Erika of his compulsion as best he could, hoping with all his heart that she might try to understand and find enough love and compassion within herself to accept his whole person the way he was.

But Erika was shocked to the core: she found the habit disgusting and began to ridicule him. Try as he might – and he tried so hard – there was no way she could understand, nor was Gerald able to give up the habit. She absolutely refused to go on living with him, making his life a mockery, and finally kicked him out of their home, leaving him to roam London for a bedsit.

And that is how, in time, he had found his way to my house.

In his struggle to free himself of his transvestism Gerald had been to see a clairvoyant, a hypnotist, and still went once a month to see a psychologist.

In trying to be cured Gerald had made a somewhat tortuous decision; in his heart of hearts he did not wish to relinquish his transvestism, which he needed and enjoyed. It created immeasurable complications: when to dress, where to dress and with whom – if at all possible – to dress. It threatened to ruin his marriage and alienate him from his children. But the enjoyment was intense, a relaxation, a thrill, a rapture, and altogether a great deal of fun.

The clairvoyant had much to say about Gerald's marriage. On asking him to let her hold any item of his while she was giving her predictions, Gerald in his wisdom had let her hold his wedding ring! His compulsion was never mentioned, though there was plenty about a marriage on the rocks, and when he asked her outright at the end, the lady was clearly taken aback and suggested – very wisely – that he consult a professional.

The hypnotist was a different matter. His taped voice, richly modulated, boomed through my living room, deep and sonorous, lulling us into a sense of profound peace and security and immeasurable trust. But it was quite powerless to cure Gerald.

Norma the psychologist had plenty of common sense and urged Gerald to stop hiding and come out into the open. He was her first transvestite client, and she learned with him and through him. Realising how highly intelligent and capable he was, recognising his forceful personality, innate drive and masculinity, she suggested that he needed to be 'fully stretched' at his work, and that this could be of great therapeutic help to him. She also realised that there was no 'cure' for transvestism.

Taking up Norma's advice to come out into the open, Gerald, a quick and willing learner, soon started telling all and sundry about his transvestism, with unexpected results. Far from ridiculing him, some of his friends had never even heard the word and had to look it up in their dictionary.

Most people were surprised but, unable to picture anything in their minds, soon forgot about it. Most important of all, it made no difference to any of them, liking Gerald anyway for the person they knew. It gave him the feeling that he, Gerald, counted for something, even though he was deviant and not quite like most other men.

As for Norma's advice to 'stretch' himself at his work, this was easier said than done. Gerald was unhappy at his new job which did not offer him the kind of challenge that he needed. Very clever people often irritate those who are supposed to be their superiors, and as the days passed, Gerald felt increasingly frustrated at his work. And during all this time he was under an intolerable strain, worried about losing his family for good.

Driving his car back from the office late one afternoon, a desperate Gerald decided to leave his future in the lap of the gods. Life or death? Let *them* decide! Revving up his engine, accelerating to 80mph, he zoomed around the sharp corner leading to my house, narrowly missing the pavement, the parked cars and the little front gardens.

The gods decided in favour of life! But the tyre marks were there for all to see days later, a reminder of Gerald's unhappy abandonment to fate.

Listening to him I began to understand the immense importance to Gerald of his cross-dressing and sensed that a whole range of complex emotions were tied up with it. I found it difficult to fathom the sheer force of the thing: a compulsion so strong as to defy all efforts to keep home and family together, making an intelligent and purposeful man helpless to break his chains.

Trying to work things out, needing to understand, my eyes wandered casually over my own attire: crimplene slacks, thick woolly jumper, flat-heeled, laced-up shoes. And the thought flashed through my mind: if *he* cross-dressed – then was I, in fact, not doing exactly the same? If I could aid him to take his cross-dressing out of hiding, share it with him and allow him to give it an airing, who knows, perhaps it might lighten his burden?

At our next *tête-à-tête* I took the bull by the horns and told him of my idea. Gerald's eyes lit up instantly: 'I was just about to ask you the very same thing!' he said, delightedly. He could see no point in delaying – we decided to go ahead that very evening. (It was not until many months later that Gerald confessed that my suggestion had come to him as a complete surprise, but quick as ever to seize his chance, he had pretended most convincingly, putting me at my ease.)

Had I had an inkling of what lay in store for me that night I might never have had the courage to make my suggestion. There had been a vague picture in my mind of Gerald slipping on a dress and a wig, and hey-presto that would be that! Instead, he now explained to me that he would be dressing 'from the skin out', and that apart from being a transvestite he was also a fetishist and 'turned on by women's clothing, in particular by lingerie'. I began to feel uneasy, though fascinated, but as there was nothing I could do about it now I decided to let events take over.

That evening, the agreed moment having arrived, we suffered a little comic delay, my first introduction to the pattern of secrecy and hiding which was to be my lot for a whole year to follow. My latest paying guest was in the process of moving in, helped by mother, just as we were about to commence our experiment, neither of us wishing at this stage to become involved in matters as mundane as welcoming a new member to the household. Gerald had arrived in his elegant grey silk dressing gown, a memento he had appropriated from a Tokyo Hotel, carrying a largish box and several bags containing gear and wig. For what seemed an eternity we had to keep ourselves absolutely immobile, hardly daring to breathe, while I was silently and agonisingly convulsed with laughter.

At last all was clear.

Carefully laying out his silken garments on the bed before him, Gerald now got into the swing of the thing. Stripping himself completely naked, he started with the tightly laced black corselette, pulling it expertly over his smoothly shaven body and stuffing it with false breasts and hip padding, then next slipped over this a pair of shiny and frilly French knickers in black, adorned with tiny pink rosettes . . .

I stood at the far end of the room, spellbound, not daring to move.

He now eased over his long, perfect legs the sheerest black nylon stockings followed by elegant and perilously high-heeled sandals, and lastly slipped on a petticoat in bright crimson, richly laden with lace.

Seating himself in front of the mirror, he first gave

himself a really close shave, then carefully rubbed a thick layer of white clown's paste into the skin to hide any tell-tale signs of beard, and topped this with a liquid make-up base. Having so far completed everything to his utter satisfaction, he now concentrated on his eyes, first trimming and further darkening his already dark eye-brows. Opening a box packed with coloured eye-shadow, he then selected a variety of hues in dark blues, greens and ocres, smoothing them carefully over his lids, achieving a truly dramatic effect. Gerald's eyes, always so brilliant and compelling, now dominated his face completely, standing out strongly against the pallor surrounding them and reminding me of pictures I had seen of tribal gods.

Gerald now removed from a small container a pair of long, black eyelashes and glued these first to his upper, then to his lower lids; next he dubbed a small brush into the rouge to give colour to his cheekbones, then lovingly smoothed over his lips a lipstick of the brightest red.

He then turned his attention to his hands. The fingernails! Gerald opened a small container and laid out before him, inside out, ten beautifully painted red nails, each of which he now touched with a special glue. When affixed over his own wide and short fingernails they quite changed the appearance of his hands, making them look pale, slender and feminine.

The make-up stage over, Gerald slipped on a sequin-covered dress in bright scarlet, figure-hugging and showing off plenty of shapely leg. For final glamour he opened a box containing his jewellery: a pair of dangling gilt earrings were attached to his lobes, next came a gilt and pearl necklace, a couple of bracelets and a sparkling ring. A few dabs of powder and a generous splashing of scent, and it was done.

I watched from my corner of the room with bated breath. He had not finished yet! Gerald opened the large box he had brought with him and lifted out of it a dark, curly, shoulder-length wig. He turned towards me and warned, 'This is the real change.' And he was right! Up till this moment I had watched him put on female costume and make-up, but what I witnessed now was a complete transformation. The moment he slipped that wig over his full head of hair there was no trace whatever left of Gerald – before me stood a perfect woman.

She turned towards me. 'I have a *femme* name, too,' she said. 'Can you guess? It's very simple, really.'

I tried. 'Jane, Joan?'

'No,' she said, 'remember my name is Gerald.'

I pondered for a moment. 'Geraldine?' I ventured.

'Well done!' said Geraldine.

We proceeded to the living room, Geraldine seating herself on the black settee: sinking into the many-patterned cushions behind her, she looked a riot of colour. Her elegantly stockinged legs crossed and showing off just enough petticoat from beneath her red dress, she was the picture of a sexily alluring and provocative female, looking well pleased with herself.

Eyeing me from across the room where I had seated myself in safety in the remotest corner, and doubtlessly well aware of my bewilderment, Geraldine now undertook to make the first move. She started on a positive note: 'I feel absolutely superb,' she said, 'soft and feminine and on top of the world. Women are so lucky! And it is marvellous having you with me – do you think I look attractive?'

I looked at her. Where was Gerald? That loveable, handsome, sparkling Gerald whom I had spoken to only an hour ago? I could not find him anywhere. Instead I was facing a strange new creature, uncanny, incomprehensible, and somewhat sinister. True, there were certain physical resemblances, but this was a different person altogether. Attractive? In which way did she mean? Attractive to *me*?

I knew that I had to proceed cautiously. A 'No' from me or even a 'Don't know' might spell disaster. Trying to take in the person facing me I had to admit to myself, yes, she did look attractive in a way, but although I had seen this type of tarty and rather overdone female so often on the screen and occasionally in passing in real life, I had up to this moment never come face to face with one, let alone sat with one in my own front room!

I must have given her some kind of satisfactory reply for, sipping her gin-and-tonic thoughtfully and chatting lightly all the while, she suddenly leaned back, and, looking me firmly in the eye, she said, 'And now I am absolutely longing for you to seduce me *as a woman*!'

I was dumbfounded.

Yet I knew that somewhere deep inside this odd female opposite me there was Gerald, the Gerald I had come to love, hiding and crying for help. And so, hesitantly and with a pounding heart, I went towards Geraldine and seated myself next to her. 'I have never made love to a woman in all my life!' I whispered, feeling frightened and at a loss. She gave me a little smile, 'You just do to me what men do to you!' she said, meaning to be encouraging.

There was a pause.

Something warm was creeping up my skirt, groping its way ever up towards my thighs. All my instincts rallied and a sharp slap came down on the intruder, my face aglow with indignation and embarrassment. 'You see?' said Geraldine looking me in the eye, not in the least perturbed. Oh – indeed, I saw all right!

Being the exact age of Gerald's own mother I had quite missed out on the permissive society, my ideas about sex and sexual love were old-fashioned and had become encrusted in that stage through a long and frigid marriage. Some years earlier when sitting in the cinema, watching Dustin Hoffman in the seduction scene in *The Graduate*, I had actually walked out of the performance, heading for home in disgust. All my feelings had been channelled towards my children and my home, by-passing my killjoy husband, and until now I had somewhat reluctantly prepared myself for a mature middle age without the slightest prospect of fun and excitement. I had become touchy and could blush as fiercely as any old-fashioned virgin at the merest mention of intimacy between the sexes. I was crippled with inhibitions and quite definitely a prime prude.

But now – could that really be me, sitting here next to my transvestite lodger who was waiting to be seduced by me, waiting for me to make the first move? Nothing around me felt quite real tonight. It could *not* be real! And because it could not be real, it had to be a fantasy. And because I was part of that fantasy I could lean towards Geraldine, put both my hands to her face and seek her mouth with my mouth. And so, in that fantasy, the ice was broken.

To my immense relief Geraldine now displayed the same empathy and understanding which up to now I had so much admired in Gerald: responding and encouraging me, putting me under her spell, she charmed me into my role. And because I loved Gerald I found it in me to love his female counterpart, feeling somewhat strange at first, yes, but also elated and out of this world, becoming initiated now into the mysteries of Geraldine.

And so it came about that Mona made love to Geraldine, and it was sweet and tender and strange and exciting as the two of us floated ever upwards, leaving earthy earth and its cares way, way beneath us.

Yet once again, our love-making over, we came crashing down to that earth where a strange reaction awaited me: Geraldine divested herself of wig and finery with double-speed, and Gerald stormed out of the room, hostility on his face.

I, to my own great surprise, felt good. I did not feel that what we had done was wrong. What had happened only concerned the two of us, and while I had had to overcome some initial feelings of rebellion concerning Geraldine and the role she wanted me to play, she in turn had to put up with my inhibitions and my clumsiness, and so the account was squared, I felt.

The following morning I caught a brief vision of Gerald in his Japanese dressing gown. There he stood framed by the kitchen door looking flushed and happy, his eyes shining, like a young girl in the first bloom of love; it tore at my heart.

He must have decided then to make our next encounter really special, because he disappeared all day to his favourite Kensington store, spending a lot of money, equipping himself for the night to follow.

The main item he purchased that day was a stiff, vividly pink tutu in the *Come Dancing* style, the waist clinched by black silk, the whole overlaid by black netting dotted about with tiny silver stars which, when worn, stood out in a wide radius all around the body. Over this extraordinary garment Geraldine had decided to wear a soft black blouse, very *décolleté* and with full sleeves gathered at the wrists. A knee-length skirt of black satin went over the pink tutu, letting it protrude by a short length, just sufficient to allow a tantalising and provocative glimpse of its riches.

When completed by wig and heavy make-up, false eyelashes and long, purple fingernails, dangling earrings and other jewellery, the result was daunting.

Looking up at her towering above me in her stiletto heels and knowing now what was expected of me, a strong feeling of rebellion welled up inside me. If on the previous night Geraldine had looked tarty, at least she had belonged to a species of female that I could recognise. This new version of hers was grotesque.

'I am not a fetishist' I ventured meekly, rendering my protest in a way she might perhaps be able to understand. 'I am not turned on by clothing.' She looked at me, I thought, astonished. 'What turns you on then?' she wanted to know. All right, here was my chance to tell her what mattered to *me*! 'His eyes, his mouth, his hands, his voice, his naked body,' I said.

Falling in love with Gerald had been inevitable for me. A beautiful man inside and out, bursting with vitality and charm, we clicked, we could talk till the cows came home, we laughed at the same things, we understood each other without the need to explain a word, we bridged that age gap effortlessly. Frequently we would divine one another's thoughts before they were expressed, we had an extraordinary rapport, uncanny. But this? There was nothing I could possibly have in common with this odd and rather intimidating figure before me.

Later Gerald told me that he, too, was cringing inside during this crucial moment. Crucial, because for him this was a test: was he acceptable as a woman? If so, he was also acceptable as a man! Or was he unacceptable, the dregs! Was he doomed to go through life a laughing stock, forever scorned and despised by women?

Geraldine felt my doubts and my bewilderment. 'It is not going to work, is it?' she asked, her voice despondent. 'Do you realise that I have made a special effort to make myself attractive to you?'

Perhaps it was this question which decided me to go through with it and play it Geraldine's way. I had got used to adapting myself to new and difficult situations throughout my life, but here was something so different from anything I had previously experienced, so virtually out of this world – out of *my* world – rather frightening and even sinister at the time. Yet still, though all my feelings were confused and up in revolt, my mind was clear enough to remind me that Gerald was inside this weird creature, watching my every reaction, waiting to be rescued.

When Geraldine sensed that I was going to be co-operative, she turned on all her considerable versatility and charm. Not for her the quick seduction! Slowly I felt myself warming towards her.

And gradually a strange thing happened: a magic began to radiate from Geraldine, ever growing and enveloping the two of us and the space around us, transforming the old fireplace with the large mirror above and the dark red carpet beneath, the obscure shapes of the leafy plants winding downwards from their hanging baskets, the ruby coloured wine in the glasses reflecting the flicker of the candles. We listened to our favourite music, we moved softly, as under a spell.

That spell never left us all night! It remained with us over our meal, throughout our talks and our silences, Geraldine no longer weird in my eyes, but drawing me towards herself ever closer by her strange allure. It followed us into the bedroom where Geraldine once more remained Geraldine, yearning to be loved for her own sake, loved and brought to life.

Turned on by me? Or by the clothes we wore? Whatever the answer to that, it was beautiful.

Then I watched Geraldine once more strip herself down to Gerald as on the night before. This time he did not storm out of the room but seated himself by the side of the bed, naked, puffing furiously at his cigarette.

I fell asleep.

When I awoke I was on my own. It was dark. An incredible sensation had come over me: my entire body had turned into music, into a great choral Mass. Every fibre of mine vibrated in unison with the unearthly sounds, merging with them.

For a long time I lay like this, being part of heaven on earth.

We now led a strange existence. Gerald felt uneasy at having involved me in his transvestism. Once again he avoided me in the evenings but in the mornings all went on as usual. We met in strictest formality. Gerald came down together with my other paying guests, and a highly embarrassed landlady served up his breakfast before he took himself off to the City. It was difficult for me to imagine my most attractive but nevertheless very masculine lodger as the Geraldine who had shared her fantasy with me.

Then one weekend Gerald returned from a particularly unsavoury scene with his wife and, looking unhappy and tense, gave me a strict order: 'Mona, take all my female clothes and burn them!' Taken aback while quite understanding his motives, I promised to carry out his order on the following day while he was away at the office.

The next morning I went through his wardrobe with very mixed feelings. Quite aware of Gerald's agonising struggle in coming to his decision, I began to wonder: could he just simply drop 'it', never to indulge in it again, perhaps to forget about it? Having gone with him through two 'sessions', it seemed to me highly unlikely. It was not only that he was clearly under the spell of female clothing, it seemed to me the only way in which he could truly relax and express himself, and in addition to this his whole pattern of lovemaking and sex were linked to it. Not for me to reason why, I was no psychiatrist!

Still, I had made a faithful promise to carry out Gerald's orders, and so I set about sorting out his wardrobe: dresses, petticoats, French knickers, bras, suspender belts, corselettes and girdles, padding, stockings and shoes, the lot. Contemplating the items before me and not sure whether to feel sad or glad, my housewifely mind simply outraged at the idea of all these costly garments going up in flames, I proceeded instead to make two heaps: one heap for charity, the other heap for Monica.

I was deep in thought, pondering with mixed feelings

the two heaps before me on the floor when I was interrupted by the shrill sound of the telephone. It was Gerald, speaking from the office. 'Hello Mona – have you burned my clothes yet? You haven't? Well – *don't!* I'll see you later.' And with this he rang off, leaving me all alone with my confusion.

For the following weekend Gerald was invited to his old schoolfriend in the country. I had overheard him talking on the telephone, asking for a woman companion: 'Tell her, one celibate exec, early thirties . . .'

As he left I kissed him lightly on the cheek. 'Have fun, my naughty womaniser,' I smiled at him. He smiled back: 'I am going to womanise all I can!' he assured me. I waved him off.

But early on Sunday afternoon as I sat all by myself on the veranda, quietly contemplating my garden, two hands holding tumblers appeared through the patio doors, followed by Gerald. He had cut short his weekend, overcome by his need to 'dress' and to be with me. The woman his friends had procured for him had turned out to be 'a pain in the neck'.

And so we embarked on a see-saw existence, where Gerald's scruples alternated with excitement and plenty of dressing-up not only of Gerald, but also of myself, trying to make myself desirable in his eyes, always under his expert guidance.

Soon our relationship entered a new phase: Gerald had instructed me to lay out his *femme* clothing for him and to insist that he should wear them, thus shifting the initiative on to me. After all, if I made him obey my command, well then, it was not *his* fault if he was cross-dressing!

'Decisions, decisions!' How often the words were to echo around the rooms in the weeks and months to come. If they were on occasion addressed to God, they were also quite often meant for me, not so much a sigh as a command, a sign that Gerald was eager to pass on to me the task of being in charge after a day's hard work at the office. What colour garments to wear tonight? Coffee or tea? 'You decide!'

Whenever he indicated a desire for cross-dressing, and soon it was to be a daily routine after he returned from the office, I laid out the items of my choice carefully on the bed, making them look tempting, arranging them in the most attractive ways that I could devise, like an accomplished window-dresser. In choosing his outfit for the evening I eventually came to gauge his moods: if he seemed unhappy I would choose ultra-feminine and more restricting garments. If I thought he wanted a quiet, relaxing evening with me over a meal I chose something a little less elaborate, toning it down to match the occasion. If he seemed excited and in an adventurous and flamboyant frame of mind I chose his most colourful and sexy clothes, but always after a day in the office which he hated, he needed to be tightly laced into a corselette.

Still, Gerald had by no means given up the idea of stopping. From time to time he would withdraw from the scene in the hope that if he managed to abstain and change his ways he might be able to achieve a reconciliation with Erika. He longed for his children desperately. Soon I too was thrown from euphoria and excitement into depression and an excruciating feeling of abandonment and longing. I had been 'hooked' on Gerald, and I was by now thoroughly addicted to him and his ways and found myself gasping for him whenever he deprived me of his company and of his love.

Thank goodness I had a safety valve, Louisa. She was possessed of plenty of common sense, she had experience of men, knew a great deal about lovers and into her ears I poured my woes at regular intervals, whenever Gerald made a renewed effort to shed Geraldine and all that was linked with her. However, leading a safe and comfortable existence as the adored wife of a model husband, Louisa found it quite impossible to fathom the extraordinary complexities of my unusual young lover when I finally spilled the secret. Her mind boggled, and there were moments, I am sure, when she suspected me of being a little deranged, making it all up.

'It is as if I have a switch behind my ear which I can turn on and off, as I like,' Gerald informed me one night as he stood before the mirror in the process of change-over, being neither wholly Gerald nor yet Geraldine. 'I can become Geraldine at any time I wish.'

Gerald, my very own enigma! I eyed him with amazement, and more than that. I envied him. Here he was, a deeply stricken man who had just lost everything in the whole world dear to him; how was it possible, I wondered, for him to become another person altogether by simply changing his *clothing*? Was it an actor's trick? I tried it out on myself by dressing up in Geraldine's most eccentric garments. True, I did feel different, adventurous and more daring, but I was still me! No escape lay that way. He must be blessed with a special gift, I thought, remembering the days when I had been a woman in trousers: I had not felt masculine. So whatever was it that triggered off in Gerald this complete transformation?

I was thoroughly bewildered by this strange phenomenon with which I now lived. Bewildered, fascinated, and intrigued. I scanned the libraries for books on transvestism, dual sexuality, transsexualism, anything that could throw light on the subject, but it appeared that not even the professionals had come up with a clue, and this included an eminent psychiatrist, himself a transvestite. It seems that the transvestite himself does not wish to be examined, he is quite happy thank you, he does not wish to be changed, does not want to have his fun analysed away, he'd rather hide and indulge furtively – but indulge he will. Most of the few who seek help have been sent by their wives who hope that their husbands may achieve a 'cure', and these are only the tip of the iceberg. The others remain in hiding, changing into their *femme* alter-egos in cars, rented accommodation, or while their families are out of the way. The compulsion has existed throughout the ages, in all cultures, enabling men to play dual roles (the ideal spy!). For compulsion it surely is.

One author writing about the history of cross-dressing tells us that transvestism is not only accepted but an integral part of many cultures and religions, playing an important part in many rites, that it is a factor deeply steeped in human development. And what about our own Western church dignitaries, I thought – the priests, the bishops, the cardinals, all in their own colourful robes, and even the Pope, wearing his virginal white one?

There are African and Indian tribes who venerate the cross-dresser as one with knowledge of both worlds, with extra perception. In Japan there is the tradition of the Noh plays and there, as well as in other Far Eastern countries, transvestism is not regarded as anything unnatural.

It is only in our Western societies that the transvestite has been rejected and ridiculed, that he has been reduced to guilt feelings and self-hatred, ashamed of something which is an integral part of his being.

And I read with a feeling of revulsion that in the not too recent past transvestites had been submitted to the horrors of aversion therapy in the shape of various forms of mental and physical torture and had even been executed.

I read that cross-dressing is the transvestite's addiction, his hobby, his drug, his adventure, his fun, his escape into a nicer and softer world. It is the butterfly he is chasing – it's what keeps him sane in a world of male pressure and demands. Off he soars into his soft and silky heaven to leave his burdens behind and become a nicer, happier, and more contented person.

I could understand this well since I too, being a close accomplice, had become caught up in it. Once involved I found myself as on a drug, floating happily in a world of allure, myth and glamour, leaving all my chains behind, soaring ever higher towards that world of scent and silky abandon of music and laughter, glitter and exotica.

From another source, the psychiatrist who was himself a transvestite, I learned that many merely needed to cross-dress in order to relax, and that sex apparently did not come into it; these would not dream of taking their 'hobby' as far as the bedroom, they had not the need.

If the transvestite was lucky and his wife accepted his cross-dressing he would make the most wonderfully devoted husband, his wife never needed to fear that he would look elsewhere for diversion. Her husband's cross-dressing fulfilled such a deep need, made him so contented, that to be able to share it with her was the greatest happiness that he could think of.

Gerald, being a fetishist for lingerie, turned on by it, had a different nature, different needs. He had little wish to make love to a woman unadorned. The naked body held no great charms for him, all mysteries revealed.

He, that extreme example of a transvestite with whom I had fallen in love, certainly bore witness to the theory of extra sensitivity. Right now he was thwarted in all his ambitions, unable to function either in family or career, and all his powers of creativity, his imagination and flair, found a perfect outlet in his transvestite activities, which he could now carry out in the setting of a normal home, and with my own full cooperation.

Until we had become lovers Gerald had existed as a 'closet transvestite'. Sometimes when he was particularly distressed he would work himself into a frenzy, as on the occasion when he had sat up all night painting his fingernails until the early hours, perfecting and perfecting and perfecting them yet again until they were the smoothest of smooth and glossy purple.

There behind closed doors he had created for himself the most glamorous and sexy female he was able to achieve, complete with false eyelashes, tarty make-up and clothing, the sexiest underwear, then turned himself on by his own creation, Gerald creating a Geraldine whom he could admire and desire in the mirror before him, thus culminating in a strange introverted sexual union. Geraldine in rapture – Gerald *in extremis*!

Let me describe Geraldine to you as she was then: she was tall and beautifully proportioned; long, dark, curly hair fell down to her shoulders, softly framing her oval-shaped face, the radiant black eyes surrounded by long black lashes, the finely chiselled nose, the expressive mouth. One curl fell flatteringly over her forehead, giving the face a soft and luxuriant appearance. The chin was firm and well-shaped, the neckline smooth, and her shoulders strong and well rounded. Her arms were perfectly formed, enhancing any sleeveless dress she may have cared to wear.

The full breasts were beautifully shaped, her waistline was very slim and she made the most of it by wearing a girdle or corselette (and perhaps a padding to achieve the desired pear-shape she considered ultra-feminine).

Her long and unblemished legs looked stunning in sheer stockings and were further enhanced by her wearing elegant and very high-heeled shoes.

She always chose very feminine garments, soft and smooth to the touch, setting off her figure to the utmost advantage. She liked to wear earrings and a necklace, a bracelet or two and rings, also a ladies' watch to complete the picture, and she always smelled beautifully.

As you looked at her you saw a perfectly shaped female, stunningly attractive in face, body and demeanour. Geraldine moved harmoniously, slowly and sensually, and she communicated a sense of calm and confidence and inner peace.

'I am taking you out of your world!' Gerald said to me one day as we sat together over lunch. He was frowning a little, worried about what he was doing to me, but I laughed in his face, amused: 'You can't do that!' I said.

He still looked doubtful, but also a little relieved, not

needing to feel so guilty, but still needing reassurance. 'Why not?' he asked, wondering at my confidence.

'Because I am far too deeply steeped in my own world. You can't take that away.' Enjoy myself I would, but my world would still be there, that ground under my feet would never give!

How little I knew. All my instincts betrayed me at that moment. And yet, how could I possibly have foreseen that other fascinating world, that world which I had only just begun to glimpse, that world which was eventually to claim me and hold me fast, spellbound?

III

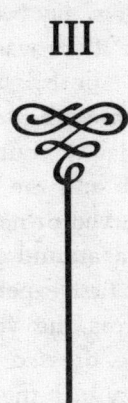

'Would you like to go to the Pembrook tonight?' asked Geraldine one day. I jumped at the idea. Geraldine had gone there once recently before teaming up with me, and I could not wait to see what it was like, and to meet up with other transvestites.

The Pembrook is a hotel where transvestites and other parts of humanity on the fringe of society can congregate freely. Geraldine in her sequined scarlet dress, meticulously made up and manicured, got us there late at night by doing 110mph in her company car, an exhilarating experience for me! She looked radiant and was in a flamboyant mood that night.

The Pembrook, situated in a distinguished Victorian crescent not far from Earls Court and reminiscent of a stately and more affluent clientele, welcomed us with a well-lit hall and a smiling receptionist who never turned a hair over Geraldine. Downstairs in a confined space dominated by the bar was a conglomeration of characters: several transvestites, gay boys, two or three girls. The din from the little disco was earsplitting, making conversation difficult. The bright lights flashed on – off – on – off, in rhythm with the din.

Jim, the barman, a lanky young fellow with a stoic expression on his face and the resigned eyes of one who had seen it all, served drinks swiftly and silently.

Surveying the scene around me, I felt excited. So this was 'it', my very first experience of mixing with transvestites. There was the young 'lady' with the sweet and gentle smile, dressed very simply in blouse and skirt, looking every inch the modern young mum; the six-footer in tight mini-skirt, exposing 'her' knobbly knees, her long face suntanned and rugged and ending in a square and prominent chin, the whole more in keeping with the looks of a macho ski-instructor of the French Alps than a female. The graceful and beautiful blonde in flouncy pastel shades showing off her long and well-shaped legs, who turned out to be a bank manager. Little Anne in low-cut flowery cotton dress who had been kicked out by 'her' wife and who had spent the past month sleeping in the back of a lorry. The drag queens dotted about the bar, ample bosoms, rich bushy wigs surrounding their heads like mobile haloes, earrings dangling, glamorously made up and wearing long, elaborate gowns and sparkling jewellery, handbags suspended from their wrists.

I noticed a great variety of types, from the exaggeratedly glamorous to the quietly dressed, talking among themselves in a corner, simple wigs and not much make-up. Most of these wore wedding rings.

Geraldine looked truly stunning that night, her eyes sparkling, knowing herself to be beautiful and attracting attention. I felt proud of her. Some of the serious-eyed young men from the far corner where the group of gays had crowded together, seeing me in the company of Geraldine, scrutinised me questioningly as if to ask, 'What are *you* doing here – are you straight, or what?' In fact this is the very question I was asked by Valerie, a tall and very slender, fragile looking transvestite who reminded me of a figurine made of precious porcelain: so delicate and finely structured and very pale, her features sensitive and sensual. To her question I could only reply in a disappointing affirmative, to which she responded that if I was Geraldine's friend I would at the very least have to wear a corselette or suspender belt! Feeling I belonged, I was very happy to tell Valerie that yes, I did.

I watched Valerie and Geraldine chatting side by side at the bar, the fragile blonde and the full-blooded brunette. It seemed that Valerie, too, had been through the excruciating ordeal of a marriage break-up as a result of her transvestism, and now she was living in female clothing practically full-time, but showed no desire to change sex, and she still loved women.

Later I saw Valerie having her hair combed: she was reclining backwards in her seat, eyes closed, her beautiful long fair hair – her own – caressed by hand and comb, every pore of her slender body enjoying the sensation, an expression of deep sensual pleasure on her face, her mouth smiling.

A wonderful feeling of freedom and total relaxation

had come over me. In these surroundings one could just be oneself, even 'straight' if that is what one was, and no one minded. You could also be as deviant as you liked if that is what made you happy, there was no one to censor or sneer. I felt a warm sensation as if sitting in a hot bath, utterly at peace with myself and my environment, feeling a horrendous weight being lifted off my shoulders, forgetting the crippling taboos that had been my lot for the past twenty years, just allowing myself to be myself.

In the meantime Geraldine had attracted the attentions of a tall, goodlooking man from the group of the homosexuals. I watched them chat together intently for a long time. The man, so I learned later, complimented Geraldine on her beauty, telling her how attractive he found her, then invited her to his house. A proposal! He promised a perfect setting: soft music and romantic lighting, a seductive atmosphere, no hurrying. He then asked Geraldine for her telephone number – mine – and promised to ring her in the next day or two.

Geraldine was euphoric. She had gone out to attract, and she had succeeded! For her that night this man's proposal was the convincing proof of her seductive charms as a woman. She felt elated, over the moon. The expression of triumph which had come over her face during the proposal never left her during our race home – another 110mph over the bridge – and stayed with her all night, as she ignored my presence. Flinging herself on arrival into the most comfortable chair, leaning backwards, her long legs stretched out before her, she concentrated on her gin and tonic, puffing smoke into the air, carried away by visions of victory and success.

What had happened? Apparently something extraordinary, something which excluded me and made me superfluous. I watched her from across the room: reclining with that triumphant expression, a superior smile on her face, she was in a pink cloud all her own, and she did not want to share it with me . . .

Next morning at breakfast a very subdued and worried-looking Gerald appeared. He had not been able to sleep all night, he had tossed and turned, tortured by doubts about his sexuality. Was it possible that he was bisexual?

Several days went by and the expected telephone call never came. Geraldine's suitor, away from the erotic atmosphere of the Pembrook, had clearly had second thoughts about the proposed romance.

However, this was not the end of the matter for Gerald. Torn by fears and doubts about his masculinity, unable to find the answer on his own and unbeknown to me, he decided to go and find out about his true nature. Several days went by while he kept himself to himself and away from me, while I felt desolate, yearning for him, craving his company, sensing that something was up.

What was up, was that Gerald went to visit a 'professional lady' as he called her, to help him find out. He wrote down his programme for her: to be dressed as a female by her, he desired a sexual encounter with another male, as an experiment. If it failed he was to be punished by the lady, dressed up by her as a maid, made to work for his mistress, and finally be subdued by her.

Suzie the lady in question, knew what she was about.

On reading Gerald's instructions she produced a black, tightly-laced corselette of very superior quality, a clinging and very shiny black mini-dress with wide silver belt to match, and black net-stockings topped by a crimson garter. Gerald had brought along his own wig. Suzie made up his face skilfully, enhancing the cheekbones to advantage and creating a sleek, tarty and very sexy Geraldine. The photographs Gerald gave me later show him as Geraldine reclining on Suzie's mauve-flowered couch in various poses of sensual allure or preening herself before the mirror, or descending Suzie's staircase, one hand slightly lifting a corner of her mini-skirt, coyly revealing net-stockings, red garter, and thigh.

After this Suzie led Geraldine to another room where she introduced her to her partner, homosexual and hooked on transvestites . . .

Geraldine did persevere through to the end, though she disliked the experience intensely. It must have been a much relieved Geraldine who was then led away by her mistress, to be redressed as a maid complete with cap and apron, to be made to work, to be reprimanded and punished. Thankfully, Geraldine knew what she was doing. She did not have direct sex with Suzie, who gave her hand-manipulation instead, while whispering titillations into her ear. There must have been a kindly soul inside Suzie. As Geraldine came, she murmured: 'There – there, is that better?' I know, I heard their tape.

Gerald had cleared up his problem in one swoop, at the mere cost of £50.

Our love affair was now allowed to flow freely, more or less, though the basic pattern remained unchanged. We were getting more and more involved with one another, often spending whole days together. There was friendship, companionship, romance, sex – not necessarily in that order – we shared his transvestism, we shared everything. Geraldine was my dream lover, as she was my dream mistress. Full of tenderness and sweetness, her generous personality enveloping me in a cloud of well-being such as I had never experienced in my life before. I no longer minded the outer changes of this lover of mine: I revelled in the variety and spice of the transvestite scene, I accepted the changes of personality that went with it, I was utterly captivated by it all.

I had come to love Geraldine every bit as much as I loved Gerald, and I absolutely adored Gerry. Gerry, my favourite: a wigless Geraldine, thus allowing me access to his beautiful dark head of hair, adorned in the most colourful and sexy garments and topped by see-through negligée or dolly nightie, jewellery sparkling from neck, wrist and ears and presenting a fantastic and exotic whole, Gerry was the embodiment of all the good things to come. I loved Gerald most of all in this in-between stage: romantic, passionate, inspired, yet utterly male in movement, gesture and in love, his beautiful eyes further enhanced by deep eye-shadow, Gerry was a creature of mystery and eroticism.

Geraldine or Gerry, both of them great romantics, would lead up to the great climax in grand style, starting from the moment Gerald returned from his office or at weekends as soon as he got out of bed. I too had to play my part. Geraldine or Gerry liked to see me wearing girdle or corselette, or else suspender belts and sheer stockings. I had got used to wearing high heels, I was learning to use make-up. The excitement and fun went on all day and throughout the evening, often until well past midnight. We always had soft music going for us, and on warm days would overflow on to the veranda, praying that the neighbours were oblivious of our strange apparel.

And yet, however beautiful our days and nights – it was invariably a hostile Gerald who left me in the early hours of the morning. Often at the breakfast table he could not bring himself to look me in the eye; the meal over he dashed out of the house, slamming the door behind him without so much as a glance backwards for a civil goodbye. It was more than flesh and blood could stand.

I decided to have it out with him.

The next time he tried to make his hurried exit I grabbed him by the arm: 'Come on, Gerald,' I said, perturbed, 'what is the matter? Why all this running away and the hostility? Have I done something wrong?'

Gerald uttered one word only: 'Guilt,' he said, and fled.

Guilt? I was amazed. Why on earth? We were two consenting adults, neither of us had any current commitment to another, Gerald having been kicked out of his home by Erika, I being independent and accountable to no one.

Gerald was very much a family man, he loved his wife and children with all his heart; they were his lifeblood. And yet – and yet he was unable to give up his cross-dressing, though God only knew he had tried hard enough, had burned his *femme* clothing more than once in the past, had been a normal husband and father for many years. But Erika demanded of him a complete repentance, she could not for one moment tolerate the thought of Gerald being dressed as a woman, and so he felt the guilt, and it crushed him.

He also felt guilty towards me. He had been drawn towards me almost from the start. I was his landlady, we had this great rapport between us, and there was physical attraction. Our age gap made it impossible for him to include me in his plans for the future, yet he had involved me in the transvestite scene, needing a partner if he was to leave the closet transvestite behind. Like all transvestites he had been dreaming of a partner for many, many years, ever since he had first dressed in his mother's bedroom as a boy. Now he had found his chance with me. He enjoyed our mutual experiences enormously, but his feelings of guilt grew and grew.

It was like the two sides of a pair of scales: his intense enjoyment of our shared experiences on the one side, the guilt feelings which inevitably followed on the other. Their weight was equal, neither outweighing the other.

My heart went out to him. Not to be able to enjoy happiness without suffering the retaliation of guilt, it seemed to me that Gerald was doomed to live between rapture and torture. When the most primitive creature on earth is entitled to its share of pleasure, why should he, so selfless, so decent and sensitive – why should he be denied that basic happiness?

I suspected that there was also one other reason why Gerald felt guilty towards me: our relationship was deepening. We both had the greatest respect for one another, knowing the other to be warm, responsible, intelligent; both of us were great individualists. With a coming together of two strong personalities such as ours the result had to be either sparks flying or the perfect merger. Having developed these feelings for me, yet burdened with the agonising suspicion that he was using me, he could not reconcile the relationship with his principles.

As for myself, our relationship was the most exciting thing that had happened to me, ever. I loved every moment of it, lived on a permanent 'high'. He was giving me so much – how could he feel guilty towards me when he was the cause of so much happiness?

If I could get this truth across to him, really convince him, surely it would eradicate his guilt feelings towards me? And if I could help him to accept himself, his *whole* self, accept his transvestism and enjoy it and see it as a source of happiness and relaxation, a kind of temporary opting out of his stressful existence as a man, surely there was nothing wrong with that? It was a great deal better than drink or drugs or crime, or any other vices that are used for just such a purpose. There is a building in my area which I pass from time to time. On a wall someone has painted in large letters:

TRANSVESTITE FUN.

And that is what it is all about.

Wanting to know more about my past, Gerald one day asked me about the man who had been my husband. I hesitated, finding it difficult to make the transition from Gerald to my former humiliation and drabness, to the man who had treated me with less respect than he had the desk in his study.

'Snob' was the first word that sprung to my mind. My ex had been a snob for a degree or anyone with an academic title. Once you had it you were Somebody, but without it you just did not count. That had put me with my unfinished education at the bottom of the ladder. It had allowed him to consider himself towering high above me in stature, a most gratifying feeling as far as he was concerned.

'Lack of humour' was the next thing. The man couldn't laugh except at his own jokes, always much to the surprise of anyone else around.

'Pessimist' was another one. He saw life in blacks and greys. Destruction, doom all around us. On a bright sunny day he was sure to detect a black cloud on the horizon. It had made life joyless.

'Mean' was the next one. I remembered only too well all those sleepless nights when I had tossed about in bed, trying to work out how to get through a week on my tiny budget.

And he was paranoid, always on the defensive, hitting back. 'Don't let me go on, Gerald, I shall become depressed!'

Gerald was quiet for a few moments, thinking. Then he said: 'I've got him – His Grey Eminence!'

It was so accurate, it made me gasp.

I had emerged, thumbs up, from a long marriage of emotional barrenness, a whole desert of it in fact, to a man who had turned out to lack everything that I valued most: sensitivity, compassion, generosity, and worst of all, a sense of humour; a man who could only ever say 'I' when it should have been 'we', who could muster warmth only for himself, a man who, in spite of an excellent salary as head of a college department was so mean I spent sleepless nights wondering how to keep the family fed and clothed, forcing me to go to him a-begging. A man who was so frigid, I sometimes thought I must have conceived his children by remote control or just by sheer luck on those rare occasions when he felt his loins astir.

In our safe detached house in suburbia I had been a model housewife, the pride of the neighbours with my well tended front garden and the shiny paintwork. I turned all my attention to house and children, cleaned and polished everything until it all sparkled and shone, children included. I must have been the most efficient slave ever, decorating and gardening, washing, cooking, bottling and baking until I had not a single moment left to myself in which to reflect.

I doted on my children, all three of them beautiful, I immersed myself in them to the exclusion of all else, allowing my maternal feelings to take over; they fulfilled me completely, and for the next twenty years or so I existed for them only. And especially for Daniel.

Daniel showed early signs of being a wonder boy. Highly intelligent and full of a delightful sense of humour, he was a musical prodigy, but he was early on rejected by his peers, and for a long time I never knew why. Endowed with a sixth sense of knowing what others felt, highly sensitive and compassionate, with enormous charm, he turned out to be a borderline autistic, preferring being beaten up to being lonely. When Daniel was ten years old or so he began to write essays full of homicidal ideas, of men drowning in submarines, of them choking to death in space ships, and always with one little man somewhere in a corner remaining alive, laughing. Himself? It was eerie – where *did* he get these horrible ideas from, he who had been surrounded with my love from the moment he was born? Fully aware of his handicap, there was no way I could shield Daniel from the horrors of his own isolation and despair. In the end my lovely boy had to go and live in a psychiatric hospital, rendered practically inanimate, though in the end he was rescued by kindly people with whom he has found a new life. At the time it nearly cost me my sanity, the pain was so great, and as always I turned to nature to regain my strength. I needed to go on, I had my two other children.

It gave me an insight into the abysmal depth and

complexity of the human mind which I could have gained in no other way, and the effort needed for my own survival had made me strong. It had steeled me.

For the years to come I banged my head against one wall or another, trying to find a way out for Daniel, a heavy grey cloud hanging over everything I did, suppressing any yearning for a little fun, for a glimpse of the lighter side of life.

We had little social life, the man who was my husband preferring his own company to that of anyone else, even that of his own family. He left Daniel for me to cope with. A cold man, swollen with self-importance, I was horrified to watch him reveal one unpleasant aspect of his character after another, until I found myself utterly repelled by him.

Loneliness threatened my life like a blight. Once the children went to school I befriended a few other mothers and we met and talked about children and teachers, endlessly. When they talked about their men, I felt left out.

No, that husband of mine had more important things to do than spend his time with us. He was the great scientist, and he was busy saving mankind, as he kept telling me. His views on how society should be run were very strict. While he spent his time at meetings I worked like one possessed taking care of house and children, giving special attention to Daniel, himself a full-time job, not to mention the huge garden, my hands plunged deep into the soothing soil. But all that did not count in the scheme of things. On the day of our final parting he told me, 'Fancy spending your life bringing up children!' And the sardonic expression on his face still haunts me to this day.

Even so, I willed myself not to leave him until the last of the children had grown up and was ready to leave home, such as it was. By that time the atmosphere had become so poisoned that I needed to leave the house as often as I could to rest my weary spirit, trying to recoup for a while.

When we were left alone in the large house it was a signal for me to petition for divorce. I shall never forget the face of the man who had been my husband for so long when I broke the news to him. He looked at me, eyes and mouth distorted with sarcasm: 'You would never dare to divorce *me*!' he said. Well, he was in for a surprise. His superb slave showed a will of her own, and two years of tough battle later managed to get her divorce, her freedom, and a new life.

The basis for my new life was a dilapidated Victorian house on the verge of collapse, which had sent all previous hopeful buyers fleeing from it in horror. But around the corner was the river Thames in all its idyllic loveliness, the swans, the ducks and the riverside cafés. I settled for it and for a while I found it hard to believe that I was now free – free from hassle, free from stress, free as a bird, to dream and to act as I wished and no one there to shatter those dreams and curb my every action. My heart leapt with relief each time I entered through my new front door, tension-free. I may have lived in a ruin and in total chaos, but the builders were there, busy, confident, and singing. The day my new home was completed we celebrated with a bottle of champagne. I had a roof over my head and a small plot for a garden, a wholly new base from which to start afresh.

When Gerald told me one Sunday morning over breakfast of the Beaumont Society, I at once suggested to him that we should join.

The Beaumont Society, it appeared, aims at helping transvestites and transsexuals with their problems of isolation, their marriage problems, and it also assists with research into this most puzzling of human compulsions.

I was enthusiastic. 'Marvellous!' I said to Gerald, 'maybe one day they will find out what makes people like yourself behave in this way. And just think, we'll be able to meet many more transvestites and find out all about them.' We could not wait to be involved and to help.

And so, together, Gerald and I worded a letter explaining about ourselves, offering our joint membership to the Society, he as a transvestite, I as his partner.

We lived in hope!

And yet – had we only known it – the Transvestite/ranssexual Support Group of London, a registered charity, was accessible to us all along, complete with counselling services, helpful literature and plenty of social activities, with an answerphone operating round the clock.

Of course I had not gone through life without hearing about the world of sexual deviances – now I came face to face with it. Gerald and I did not visit the Pembrook often, but whenever we did I had a chance to meet people from this other, fringe, world, until recently so firmly closed to me. These people were real, not just sensational paragraphs in the more popular press, which in any case I had rarely read. Here, in this place, I found myself talking to them. Wendy, whom we had discovered tonight, was a rough diamond, her manner of speech as direct and unpolished as could possibly be. If she referred to her penis as 'dick' and the breasts she was waiting to have installed as 'boobs' that was OK, as descriptive as anything. She was open, frank and earthy, and without the slightest trace of pretence. I liked her. I felt sure Wendy was kind-hearted and would put herself out for a friend or anyone she felt deserving of her help and sympathy.

Wendy was male, gay, and dressed in female garb. Her off-the-shoulder dress accentuated her long neck which tonight was adorned with a double pearl-choker, with bracelet to match. Her high heels made her rather tall, and she carried herself well. As yet she was flat-chested, but in eight weeks' time precisely she was going to have her pair of 'boobs' installed at a

Harley Street Clinic, and she simply could not wait for the event to happen. Boobs! She was then going to pass more easily as a proper female, but intended to leave her lower parts intact, being very proud of her 'dick', while loving men as sex partners. She made no attempts at all to disguise her booming masculine voice, which she now used to explain to me that she could well understand heterosexuals, homosexuals (of course!) and lesbians. 'But I just cannot understand bisexuals,' she exclaimed, emphasising the point with her constantly moving hands, 'I just cannot understand them!'

I wondered at this. When Wendy was going to have her 'boobs' installed in two months' time, what was she going to be if not to all intents and purposes a hermaphrodite, the very symbol of the condition she told me she could not understand? Oh well! I was learning to accept people as they were, and I did not argue with Wendy about her apparent lack of logic, as she seemed to be so very content with her lot and her way of looking at people.

Wendy worked for herself as a beautician from her own flat, and I felt certain that her lady clients liked her enormously, and that she provided them with a glimpse of light-heartedness and unpretentiousness which they lacked in their everyday life.

She hoped fervently that once she was the proud owner of boobs she would be able to find a permanent partner, a constant companion. 'I am well into my thirties now,' she said, 'and I do not wish to spend the rest of my life living on my own!'

I thought, 'I cross my fingers for you, Wendy!'

At the bar sat Caryn. Tall, dark and vivacious, in a tight black velveteen dress and sparkling gold ear-rings below her softly coiffured wig, she nevertheless revealed the well-groomed features and demeanour of the successful public-school-educated businessman. Caryn, who resided in Mayfair, had spent the better part of the week in the directors' boardroom.

'I sit there in my pinstripes with the tie and briefcase, and underneath I am wearing the silkiest, frilliest under-wear. It makes me feel good, it caresses my body. I like to think that I have this secret and inside I'm laughing – if only you knew!'

Caryn had an accepting girlfriend. 'She knows that I would never give it up, not for anyone, not even for her, not after all *I've* been through.'

My eyes now roamed over an animated foursome of females in the far corner, seated around a table. One young woman in particular caught my attention: long, sleek chestnut hair fell softly down to below her shoulders and on to her long white dress, her low neckline framed in a sparkle of gold. With lovely features, huge dark eyes, a small delicate nose and full red mouth, she was petite and exquisitely slender, with an ethereal beauty that I could not but envy her.

She said something that I did not catch and then, unhurriedly, lowered one white shoulder of her dress and proudly revealed a most perfect young breast to the exclamations and sincere admiration of her friends.

Later I learned that the beauty was in fact Linda, a male transsexual – on hormone treatment for some time, but not yet operated on . . .

At the far end of the bar sat a group of middle-aged housewives, deep in conversation. Dressed very quietly, wearing simple blouse and skirt or a neat day dress, with minimal jewellery, they were utterly convincing in everything but their voices. After a couple of Martinis I managed enough courage to edge my way towards them, eager to satisfy my curiosity. 'Joyce' turned out to be an American, over in London on one of her regular business trips, married with three children. Did her wife know? 'Oh Gawd no,' was the answer, 'she would never understand!' So how did Joyce cope? 'I just dress whenever I get the chance,' she said, 'I stay at the Pembrook when I come over, I do all my *femme* shopping here, which is absolutely great, I usually do it as Joyce, I enjoy myself, I relax. At home it's back to realities.' The other two, Peggy and Sophie, were Londoners. Peggy's wife 'probably knew', but turned the other way. Sophie's wife 'had no idea'. I was amazed when I heard that both of them transformed themselves regularly in their cars. What an extraordinary feat of acrobatics!

Geraldine and I were in conversation with Nina, on leave from an oil rig. Nina was a drag queen, heavily made up and bejewelled, her wig surrounding her head in a huge fuzzy copper bush, overshadowing her face which did not fit: it was heavy and male and not attractive. I felt sorry for her, I was sure that she must be unattractive even as a man. Nina wore a long, pink and grey dress, heavily embroidered with sequins, her skirt widening out from the waist down to her feet, which were encased in narrow and perilously high-heeled evening shoes made from the same material as the dress, and her evening bag too was matching. It seemed the oil rig was yielding good money for Nina.

We talked to her for an age, but Nina never strayed for a moment from the topic of her work on the oil rig. I was deeply impressed by the detailed description of her knowledge and manifold skills, but Geraldine said, 'Why go to all that trouble to make yourself feminine, if you then spend the entire evening trying to convince people how masculine you really are?'

For the following Saturday we had planned an outing to Barkers of Kensington, Gerald's favourite store, which catered for all his needs. Well, practically all. There were a few items he got from Ma Cutler's little shop in Islington which stocks all the requirements to satisfy its transvestite customers: size 12 shoes with 6-inch heels, for instance, false breasts, sexy corselettes, French maids' outfits, and lots more. And of course any amount of transvestite magazines and fantasy stories.

But today it was Barkers, where Gerald had discovered Larry, who supplied him with wigs. Larry turned out to be a mild-mannered young man, and he and Gerald were on splendid terms. I remained with them in the cubicle while Gerald tried on his wig, which was in need of being redressed. It was a strange sight that met my eyes: Gerald correctly suited and completely male was trying on his long, curly wig – the body of

Gerald topped by the head of Geraldine. Larry arranged and rearranged the curls on Gerald's head this way and that, his skilled, clever fingers knew exactly what they were about. Checking and re-checking in the mirror before them, Larry listened carefully to Gerald's suggestions until they were both happy with the results and Gerald's head was much enriched with curls.

Now Gerald's eyes lit up as he had one of his spurts of impulsive generosity. 'Let's have a wig for Mona!' he exclaimed. My heart sank. My hair, cut very short as it was, did not please him: he would have liked it to be long, curly and feminine. I was beginning to wish that the floorboards would swallow me up, and I felt embarrassed before Larry.

If I had felt uneasy before, watching this bizarre session, I was near to panic now that I was going to be the centre of their attention, but Gerald looked so full of enthusiasm that I sat myself meekly before the mirror to comply with his wishes. A succession of different wigs were tried out on my head: brown, auburn, black, wavy, curly, parted on the left, parted on the right, medium long, very long, and I felt terrible in all of them. After a lot of deliberation we finally made our decision: auburn curls and medium long. We stuffed it all into a box, thanked Larry profusely, and took our leave.

On we went now to the lingerie department. Gerald headed first of all for the counter selling girdles and corselettes. I felt inhibited by Gerald's presence – this was my first experience of shopping for *femme* items with him – the situation was unusual and I resigned myself to watching him handle the garments on the display tables, lovingly testing and feeling each one for quality, workmanship, material, shape and the sheer pleasure of it: he was an expert on female underwear. Occasionally he turned to me for my opinion, but alas, with poor results. I had never worn a corselette or girdle until meeting him! He was quite clearly disappointed not to have my active participation, but I felt the scene to be a strange one. It was I who was the fish out of water, while he was obviously thoroughly at home, our roles reversed. After making the most of touching and testing, he finally made his purchases: a black corselette for me, a white bra and several pairs of frilly knickers for himself . . .

If Gerald was rapidly making me a part of his fantasy world, I in turn felt it was time that I introduced my lover to the finer side of life, to acquaint this businessman whose brains revolved round production lines, profits and losses, etc. with the joys of the arts. I knew he loved music – we were never without it – but it appeared that although Gerald was a man of the world and had travelled all over the globe, he had never once attended a live concert. I therefore betook myself to the Albert Hall to book two seats for a promenade concert, in the hope of making up for this lack, to open his mind, his ears . . . I was on a cultural mission and I looked forward to the event with the greatest anticipation.

He met me at the Albert Hall, casually dressed

and looking somewhat tense, but then I expected this since it was Gerald I was meeting and not Geraldine, and the concert hall was unfamiliar territory for him.

Our seats were fairly near the orchestra and with a good view of the players. The concert began with a piece by a contemporary composer, and I was wondering how he would like it, but I never found out: Gerald had spotted among the violins an attractive lady player, and from then on he never stopped looking at her throughout the performance. His eyes with their strange hypnotic quality glued themselves to the lady in question with such persistence that I feared he would put her off guard, making her play the wrong notes and cause a fiasco.

I watched with amusement. I felt certain that I saw her notice him and get flustered. With eyes like that – what woman wouldn't?

The interval turned out to be a relief, at least it afforded them both a break from the persistent staring, but when Mozart took over, Gerald carried on exactly where he had left off and this time I was sure I saw the lady look up from her fiddle straight at Gerald and turn a vivid colour.

When a few months later I booked for another concert I made quite certain that we did not sit too near the orchestra . . .

Today was Sunday, and after lunch Gerald changed into a particularly graceful Geraldine: virginal in her sleeveless white dress with a lace pelerine reaching almost down to her waist and with sheer white stockings and shoes, her curly black hair and the flushed, radiant face providing a lively contrast, she was gentle and in pensive mood.

Outside the elements were raging, thunder and lightning were shattering our peace. Geraldine put her arm around me and wordlessly we moved on to the patio, to feel at one with the elements of nature and to merge with them, the torrential storm roaring all around us, enveloping us. The sounds of the storm and the music inside us blended into a furious symphony, making us feel eternal yet small, and humble.

It became one of those nights of perfect harmony. Geraldine had left all her pain and tortured guilt behind with Gerald, she was sweet and relaxed and at peace with herself. Together we listened to our favourite music to match our mood: Dvorak, Mozart, and of course our special favourite, James Galway playing his Magic Flute. Tonight we did not have much need of words.

Quietly we sat over our meal with the soft music and the wine, the candlelight caressing Geraldine's face, a picture of complete purity and beauty. We opened wide the patio doors, not wishing to lose touch with the elements outside, inviting them in, the raging thunder and lightning only serving to highlight the peace within ourselves.

We had lost all touch with time, quietly we succumbed to the passing of the night. Silently in the early hours of the morning we moved into the bedroom for our loving. The storm still raged . . . and we, who had been stirred by it were overcome by an unearthly feeling of unreality and a happiness so vast it could only relate to the furies outside and sweep us away into eternity, Geraldine and me, Mona.

And before saying good night Geraldine discarded all her clothes and behold, there was naked Gerald, Adam emerging from Eve, and overcome by our mutual experience we knelt by the bed side by side, and Gerald prayed to God, crying. Prayed for forgiveness for our sins, asking God to be tolerant of one who was servant to a harmless compulsion, wanting to hurt no one, asking Him to shield and protect all his beloved ones.

Amen.

Even so, I could not help wondering sometimes: does he use me as a kind of guinea pig to test a woman's reaction to himself as a transvestite? If so, this was only to be expected and I on my part, loving him and desiring him madly, while at the same time knowing my own strength and resources and sensing all the possibilities of a continuing relationship, was quite happy to carry on.

Seeing that Gerald was also a fetishist and turned on by female clothing, in particular lingerie, I had often asked myself: does he make love to *me* or to my suspender belts? One day I tackled him outright. As usual he was perfectly honest. 'Both,' he said.

As time went on and our relationship deepened ever

more Gerald became convinced that God had guided his steps towards me and from time to time he would converse with Him and thank Him.

He also thanked me for allowing him to become what he had always longed to be, all his dreams come true. 'I have never been so happy!' he assured me again and again. And, 'You are the most important person in my whole life, Mona. I am so lucky – you are one in a million!'

It was all most encouraging and made me feel great and wonderful. Then, to make certain that the dream would continue for a long time to come, he gave me a number of strenuous exercises to do – 'To keep you fit and young for me for as long as I can'. It so happens that I am fairly good at exercising, and what greater incentive could any woman ask for?

Often Geraldine would ask me to tell her, reassure her, 'I prefer you like this – I do not want you any other way!' It worked on her like a spell, absolved her from any feelings of unease which she might have had about herself, it was her password to paradise.

It had struck me, however, that Gerald needed a great deal of verbal reassurance during lovemaking. Was he perhaps afraid of being sexually unattractive because of his transvestism? I felt I was beginning to understand this man with his strange needs and compulsions. I was by now fully participating in his transvestism; I enjoyed seeing him dressed *en femme* as Geraldine, or in his in-between state as Gerry, without a wig, usually wearing exotic underwear and see-through negligée. The whole scene as created by him was one of wonder, mysterious and magical and it lifted me right out of my ordinary everyday existence and straight up to cloud nine.

At the same time I was beginning to learn a part quite new to me: how to make myself attractive to My Man. Gerald was taking me in hand for the purpose of turning me into a female he could thoroughly approve of and desire. He instructed me to let my hair grow, lose a stone and a half in weight, wear high heels and suspender belts, girdle or corselette, and paint my fingernails a bright red, just to mention a few. All great fun, but not that easy to comply with when for an eternity you had been married to a man who had neither noticed nor cared what you wore or indeed if you wore anything at all. Occasionally I stopped to wonder what had happened to that other Monica, the one I was rapidly leaving behind: she had been both workhorse and earthmother, fond of trees and children, creatures and home-baked bread, but excitement, fun, romance or sex had not featured in her life at all.

But now I was dressing up too! Reluctantly at first and feeling rather sheepish, I soon discovered that any resistance was useless. Gerald wanted me to look sexy and feminine and if I wanted to keep him – and I did – I had to go along with him, 'Look good, smell good, feel good.'

It did not take me any time to get hooked on the scene. I had long had a yearning to become more feminine and to feel a little pampered from time to time, but I had never anticipated that one day I would have a beautiful and exciting young lover to enforce it.

I revelled in my new role. Searching the stores

for sexy underwear, scents, sprays and creams, eyeshadows and mascaras, I had one aim in mind only: how to make myself as seductive as I possibly could for my lover.

If I was enabling him to become what he had always dreamed of being, it was equally true that he did the same for me. At long last I felt myself becoming a complete woman.

Six pairs of crimplene slacks size 18 in assorted colours went by the board that early summer. I threw them away with relish, and into the dustbin with them went my prudery and inhibitions, my dowdiness and my lack of self-esteem. I might no longer be in the first flush of youth, but I could still be attractive and feminine, and I had all the proof I needed that I was still desirable. I felt on top of the world as I walked along in tight skirt and new shoes, my step much lighter, my feet barely touching the ground.

And still my lover was not satisfied with my various attempts at transforming myself for his pleasure. Earrings, it seemed, were an absolute *must*. I managed to venture a mild protest, 'What – at this stage of my life?' But he just ignored my doubts and one fine morning packed me off to Barkers and to Larry. Larry does ears as well as wigs, and in no time at all – hey presto! there was I, a couple of gold sleepers in my lobes, one step further still towards that complete sex symbol for Gerald.

I must admit that it took me no time at all to enthuse about my reflection in the mirror with my new ornaments. So much so that I felt positively naked when leaving them off. It all just goes to show!

The thought occurred to me: was I not actually reversing the modern trend for woman's emancipation by going all out to adorn myself for the sake of mere man? Was I swimming against the stream? I did not think so, and I did not care. I had been a poor slave for far too long and a very dowdy slave at that, and no one had given a damn about my character or feelings so long as I had kept on slaving. Now I was turning myself into a liberated woman, free to live with my lover – free to live with my transvestite lover – my confidence grew with every pair of seamed stockings, high-heeled shoes and French knickers, not to mention all the other tempting garments and accessories I could and would buy, the only limitation being the contents of my purse.

IV

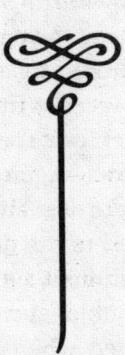

Every now and then Gerald's burdens and guilt feelings became too much for him and he felt the need to be cleansed and redeemed, and so he craved punishment much as some sinners crave for the confessional. Punishment, that is, from the hands of Dominant Woman – *me*?

Yes, me. He introduced me to the scene with gentleness and patience, trying to make me understand his needs, his eyes and voice persuasive, while I trembled at the prospect before me. Because I knew that I was going to comply, that there was nothing that I would not do for him. Straining to overcome my own natural feelings which were of love for him, of tenderness and compassion, I shrank from the picture he painted before me. I was aching with every fibre to soothe and caress his worries away, and causing him pain was not written into my code of behaviour.

He did not ask too much of me for this, our first rehearsal – he played it down. Listening to him carefully I began to wonder: if, by hurting his body I could at the same time remove some of the pain from his heart, then perhaps the strange procedure was justified after all? His body would soon recover from the ordeal, and his soul might perhaps achieve some measure of peace? And with this in mind I began to prepare myself for the task ahead, trying to visualize the scene awaiting me, getting myself used to his new demands on me.

Although the punishment he asked of me on this occasion was only a mild spanking, still I found it hard to do as he wished when face to face with him, waiting for his ordeal. I who had never laid a finger on my own children! There he lay spread out before me, so vulnerably naked, so defenceless, so beautiful that it took my breath away, and he longed to be chastised by my own two hands.

Tremblingly, feeling faint, I set to my task – meekly at first and only slowly growing bolder. The spanking I dealt him clearly caused him pain, but it also gave him pleasure, the two sensations as complementary to one another as the two sides of a single coin.

It seemed I was acquitting myself well! Gerald praised me, and he grew more ambitious. And as for me, I came to understand him a little better, gained a little more insight into the dilemmas his poor soul was lumbered with, his strange ways of dealing with them. And I had learned the rudiments of my technique.

He was now keen to act out a slightly more complex

fantasy. With much trepidation I consented to try out the scene he suggested. It appeared that Gerald longed to be my maid, to be ordered about by me, to hoover and to dust, to polish and make beds, to wash the kitchen floor. The scene was to end with my displeasure and his subsequent penalty.

On the morning in question Gerald came down the stairs in navy blue blazer and grey flannels, quiet and formal, every inch my perfect lodger. I in turn responded by being the perfect landlady: courteous, polite, reticent.

How to bridge that gap? Where to make a start?

Time dragged and became heavy. For a while it seemed as if neither of us was able to change our roles. Then, mustering all my courage, making a supreme effort, I summoned Gerald into my bedroom. There, my voice icy, I criticised his behaviour: he was a 'lousy lodger – sloppy, noisy, untidy'. If he wished to remain in my house he would have to make amends by working for me, in short, by becoming my maid.

He protested, of course, looking shaken and mumbling apologies, while I, losing no time, got hold of this indignant man, stripping him completely naked, turning a deaf ear. I now put on him my shabbiest underwear, the dowdiest cotton frock, apron and head scarf, and the only flat-heeled and open-toed sandals he could squeeze his feet into. Leaving 'her' with my explicit orders indoors I preferred to sit it out in the garden, feeling ill at ease and rather queasy, my heart pounding wildly, while indoors my new maid flitted about from room to room doing my work for me at a breathtaking speed, much more efficiently than I could ever have done, on her face an expression quite new to me: frightened, subservient, and wholly submissive.

It was my agreed task to inspect my maid at intervals and therefore, a little while later, I assumed an air of confidence and dragged myself indoors. Everything, indeed, sparkled and shone. The wooden dining table gleamed at me and so did the sink and the cooker, and right now my maid was busy polishing the kitchen tiles! Even so, it was my task to rebuke her for her shoddy work, to criticise and to scold her, and so I did not mince my words, telling her what I thought of her. An expression of great terror came into the eyes of the poor wench, and in a voice barely audible she whispered, 'Yes Madam,' and 'Sorry, Madam, it won't happen again,' after which I speedily removed myself back into the garden much in need of fresh air, relieved it was all over for the moment.

I had always enjoyed acting when a child at school and had been good at it, but this was different. Whilst I acted, he did not! He *was* that maid during our session, and any hint of pretence on my part would have ruined the show for Gerald, and turned our charade into a calamity for him.

Although my new maid rushed around so busily, exerting herself to please her mistress, when she finally came to the end of her chores asking for my approval, I had to look stern and was on no account to show satisfaction with her: did I not discover a speck of dust on the picture frame, a breadcrumb on the kitchen floor? Why had she not wiped the door handle? I was outraged, I was scathing. Was this indeed the best she could do for me? If so, she was certainly not fit to be my maid!

She looked crestfallen. She begged my forgiveness. She pleaded, she was very, very sorry. She was almost in tears, willing to atone for her shoddy work in any way I asked.

But I, speechless and furious, just pushed her. Pushed her down and on to the bed, crushing her underneath me, punishing her the only way I knew.

In playing out his fantasies with me, Gerald followed quite a deliberate course. It was all part of his coming out into the open as advised by Norma.

'I want no secret from you, Mona – I want you to know me, warts and all,' he had said to me one day, and I had felt deeply honoured at such confidence. I loved this man, and I would accept him as he was, quirks, compulsions, fantasies, the lot.

'I can feel it in my bones that you can do it,' he had assured me soon afterwards, with a view to be encouraging after telling me of some of his more unusual fantasies, while I had sat opposite him, feeling doubtful.

In the past Gerald had periodically visited prostitutes in whatever part of the world he had happened to find himself at the time, as an outlet for his needs for submission and for sex when 'dressed'. It had left him afterwards feeling guilty and uncomfortable with himself.

Now he had me.

A couple of weeks later the need for redemption was with Gerald once more. This time he absolutely longed to be an intruder in his landlady's bedroom, to be discovered in the act and punished by her severely. He programmed me minutely. As I opened my bedroom door at the appointed time this was the scene that met me: someone was moving inside! I could just make out the slim figure of a man, smart navy blue suit, dark hair – and now I could see the handsome face disfigured by a petrified expression. 'Oh, my Lord!' I exclaimed in horror as I recognised the features of my impudent lodger from upstairs. My anger rose quickly: this was the moment to assert my authority once and for all, to show this trespasser without delay what mettle I was made of, to be firm with him and make quite certain that he would never ever repeat this outrageous intrusion into my private domain.

From my culprit's terror-stricken expression it became quite obvious that he, too, was taken completely by surprise.

'What on earth are you doing in my bedroom?' I demanded, my voice seething with anger, but all he managed to utter in the way of reply was a confused and mangled stutter.

I must act quickly, I thought, put my foot down

at once, punish him and teach him a lesson he will never forget. But how?

Trying hard to keep a cool head I searched for a way. Suddenly, in a flash, I had an idea – this should do it! If I was to turn this offending man into a woman, surely this would be the best punishment of all? Quickly I got hold of this criminal and wasted no time ridding him of his beautiful dark business suit and all his underwear too, and, confronted with this stark naked and cringing male, proceeded to dress him in my most sexy, feminine garments, putting on him my girdle, bra, knickers, etc., while enjoying every moment of his humiliation. Next came the make-up. I applied eye-shadow and mascara to his eyes, foundation and blusher to his skin, lipstick to his lips, taking my time over it, drawing out each stage for as long as I could, to make the maximum impression on my helpless victim. I chose a very sleek and feminine dress for him and finally, for the ultimate disgrace, adorned him with a long, dark, curly wig.

And now I stood back to scrutinise my creation. 'You make a perfect woman!' I told him. 'Now show me if you can move like a woman, too,' I demanded. 'Walk up and down before me – move your hips more gracefully, swing them a little!' To my great surprise he paraded himself before me splendidly, revealing the greatest aptitude.

Then I subdued him, punished him, enjoyed him, forced him to do my bidding. Why pretend? It was glorious, heaven can hold no greater bliss. He was all mine to do with as I wished.

After that Gerald felt a great release from his pressures – and it lasted for quite a while.

As for me? I felt I had not changed by doing what I had done, I was still the same person, quite sane and down to earth, our feelings of love and respect for one another were not affected, though I had learned something new about the obscurer corners of human nature, including my own.

While the bonds between us strengthened and grew, Gerald's hope of ever rejoining his family dwindled. He could see no way ahead, the future looked bleak and threatening. Crushed by pain and guilt feelings and hating himself for what he was, he could not play the game at his place of work in the way which was expected of him.

Gerald had been trained amongst other things as an economist and a market researcher. When asked one day by the company chairman of his engineering firm for an assessment of their prospects, Gerald did an honest job: he severely criticised the way the business was run, going into fine details, and finally forecast bankruptcy unless the whole policy of the company was changed, making alternative suggestions.

The chairman did not take too kindly to Gerald's bleak forecasts and took it as a personal slight on his own judgement. He developed a strong dislike for him from that moment on, and it did not take long before Gerald found himself demoted. The luxurious company car, the one which had conveyed us so swiftly to our outings at the Pembrook, was replaced by a more modest model in keeping with his newly lowered status.

Though he bravely hid the blow behind his acute sense of humour, I could nevertheless see the hurt. Gerald, cut out to be captain of the ship, was now a mere cog in the wheel and I knew that it could never work.

Gerald still visited his psychologist, Norma, regularly once a month. If he had gone initially to see her in the hope of becoming 'normal', a man like other men, of keeping home and family together, he realised now that this could not be done. He had begun to come to terms with himself, his transvestism and his fetishism, he enjoyed them enormously, and he had found me to prove that he was acceptable and loveable just as he was.

Although Norma was not able to cure him of his transvestism, she had given him good counsel from the start, he trusted her and told her about us from the very beginning of our relationship, starting with our nightly intimate talks, his confession to me and my response.

Norma had sensed that there was more to come. One day, after not having seen Gerald for some weeks she asked him straight out, 'Have you seduced your landlady yet?' He had by then, indeed! I thought she had shown great perception throughout. She had never at any time tried to eliminate Gerald's compulsion as the hypnotist had done; he was lucky with her.

One day Gerald showed Norma two photographs of himself as Geraldine. The first one pictured him in the white dress which she had worn on that unforgettable day in the rainstorm. The long, dark curls framed Geraldine's relaxed and beautiful face; she was sitting by the side of the dining table, a glass of dark red wine before her. Her arms rested lightly on the sides of the chair, her lovely long legs were clad in white stockings and shoes and crossed towards the camera, and the whole picture conveyed an atmosphere of harmony and peaceful domesticity.

The second picture showed Geraldine in the black mini-dress with the silver belt as arranged by Suzie, the professional lady. Geraldine was reclining on Suzie's bed with the mauve-flowered cover, her body was half-raised and one hand was caressing her hip, the heavily made-up eyes looked with an expression of potent sexuality down at thigh and leg in black net-stocking, just exposing a corner of the red garter. The picture, a composition in blacks, mauves and browns with the silver belt affording the only visual relief, gave one the feeling of peeping through a secret hole in the wall, just about to witness a forbidden scene.

Norma's verdict when shown the two photographs side by side was, 'The first picture shows you happy and relaxed; on the other one you are acting . . .'

In answer to Norma's question Gerald had told her that our relationship had deepened, how it allowed him to cross-dress at any time he wished, and that I fully participated in this and even helped him to play out his fantasies.

Norma said to Gerald, 'You will never be happier

than you are now, you don't need me any longer,' and with these words she dismissed him and in doing so handed him over to me.

He came home telling me the good news, his black eyes beaming at me, and I felt proud. I knew that I could 'do it', that I was in a unique position to do it, and that I would do it thoroughly and well.

It was time for me to take stock of the situation.

Looking back over the past few months and marvelling at what was happening to me, I could not help pondering about the differences between myself and the woman who was still Gerald's wife. I knew very little about Erika, it was hurtful for Gerald to talk about her, but I was well aware that she was physically everything he could desire: perfect in her slim beauty, her blonde hair and her aloof self-confidence, she was everything that Gerald was not: she was normality personified. Erika had grown up in a prim and narrow environment, the only child of well-to-do Swiss parents who doted on their beautiful daughter, cushioning her with an abundance of material comforts. For her the proof of love consisted in a diamond, a fur coat or the latest model of a washing machine. As far as I knew, Erika had never had to struggle, had had no hurdles to climb, no reason to pitch herself against her environment. She became the perfect housekeeper, an excellent cook and a good mother to their two children, and that was as far as it went. Sexually, she had not been as responsive as Gerald would have liked, needing a good deal of coaxing, cooling off easily.

As soon as Tommy, their second child was born, Erika had pressed Gerald for a vasectomy, and out of love for her he very nearly complied. He was twenty-eight years old at the time.

It seemed to me that apart from being a sister female, there was very little else I had in common with Erika.

It was only the other day that I had asked Gerald, 'If Erika, to you, stands for normality, then what do I stand for? Abnormality?' And he had smiled at me, his eyes full of love, and said, 'Not abnormality, Mona. *You* stand for love and compassion!'

If Erika had accepted her environment without asking questions, I on the other hand must have been born with doubts in my guts. One of my earliest memories is that of our lovely nanny, Berta, a devout protestant, teaching me and my little brother Maxie to fold our hands and say a prayer:

> *Lieber Gott, mach mich fromm*
> *dass ich in den Himmel komm.*

> Dear God, make me devout
> so I may enter heaven.

Young as I was, something did not seem quite right to me about that prayer. If you were not devout but still good – did you not enter heaven, did you then enter hell? Anyway, I was not going to be told one way or another, I was going to make up my own mind. Later I had irritated my well-meaning teachers by asking awkward questions, and I am pleased to think that I still ask those questions. It does not make for an easy life or for popularity either, but that's the way I am.

Pain and suffering and injustice were facts of life I had been introduced to at a very early age, coming from a Jewish family. Berlin, 1933: my brother and I stand in front of the open window of our first floor flat, listening to the boom-boom of the drums and the brass music and the singing coming towards us from behind the street corner. I turn to look at Maxie. His face is flushed with all the excitement, his eyes shining; he is a little smaller than I, he is only four. Behind us stand our parents, their faces ashen. Here they come, the strong men all in a row, all in brown: brown shirts, brown helmets, brown breeches, brown boots. As they pass beneath our window, flags flying, we can make out the words of their song quite clearly, their rhythm sharp, clipped, precise:–

*Ja, wenn das Judenblut vom Messer spritzt
Dann geht's noch mal so gut ...*

You want it translated? Watch out – it's not pretty!

> Yea, when the Jew's blood squirts from the knife
> All will go twice as well ...

And the jackboots crashing down on the pavement below.

Not a placid childhood, no. But Maxie and I were lucky to get out in time, escaping to Palestine – while our parents and nearly all our relatives stayed behind to meet their fate.

V

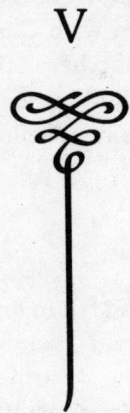

When Norma handed Gerald's well-being over to me, I knew that this was a chance in a million. What more could any woman in love ask for?

Gerald found that my reactions to his ups and downs were what he needed; he felt himself loved and respected in spite of his deviant lifestyle, I treated him as a whole and complete human being and not as a freak, and this was balm to his injured ego. He found refuge, shelter and warmth in our relationship. For me it was a time of testing: testing of my patience, my ability to adapt, to divine and forestall, to fall in with Gerald's moods and needs, and always, always, with a view to strengthening that vulnerable inner core of his.

Then one night after three months or so of our colourful and unusual romance, with both of us aware we were coming ever closer together, the incredible happened.

We had returned from the local cinema where we had watched a Western with Clint Eastwood, Gerald's ideal He-Man, his macho hero. That night, as we made love to one another leisurely, something clicked inside Gerald, matured and came to a flowering: he fell in love with me.

He?

Or was it Geraldine who fell in love with me? Throughout our romance Gerald had been keeping himself somewhat remote, being a warm and wonderful friend, fond of me, respecting and needing me, while all along realising that I could never be for him, not with the age gap so unbridgeable. For Gerald one day there would have to be a younger woman, younger and of childbearing age, who would give him the family life he so craved for.

But Geraldine was a different matter entirely. For her I could fulfill her every need, and those needs were complex, often inexplicable, and together we could explore them to their deepest possibilities. Geraldine needed me in order to become flesh and blood, to breathe and to live, to love and to be loved.

Yet Gerald was also Geraldine, as he was Gerry, their relationship a symbiotic one. I expect that this is what made him suggest the following day that he move in with me downstairs, 'to live together'.

In spite of everything Gerald's suggestion took me aback; my own memories of a shared lifestyle were traumatic. I valued my independence most highly. What is more, our love-romance was so extraordinarily beautiful, so other-worldly, so brimming over with fun and excitement, I felt it could not possibly be improved upon by any changes. And so I refused.

He took it all right, though it occurred to me later that perhaps my refusal featured as yet another rejection of himself, adding another bruise to his fragile ego.

And so Gerald remained in his little den upstairs, while we managed downstairs as before. Nevertheless, he now made ambitious plans to turn 'our' bedroom into something perfectly feminine, into 'our perfect love-nest', and he elaborated at great length as to how this might be achieved: a double-bed was the first must, a coffee table here, a comfortable chair or two there, a lamp over the bed, and he would build us a splendid dressing table. Last of all, a carpet of the deepest pile. His imagination carried him away and I listened to him with the greatest pleasure and fascination, but also with a heavy heart. It sounded all much too good to me, and anyway, how long could it all last? I could hardly believe that we had made it as far as this, though the facts stared me in the eye: my beautiful lover, there he sat by my side while I lay on the bed before him, and he eulogised by the hour about our future . . .

Meanwhile at Gerald's place of work matters went from bad to worse. Having been demoted a few weeks earlier, he now had little cheer in the tasks allotted to him. Thank goodness he had a safety valve, his escape into cross-dressing, able to shed worried Gerald and become relaxed Geraldine at any time he wished.

To boost his confidence and make the hateful office bearable he wore girdle and stockings to work each day. As the tension accelerated he relied increasingly on his cross-dressing to carry him over.

And true enough, before long Gerald was told that he was no longer needed, and he was on the dole.

Gerald on the dole! What a waste of intelligence, ability and drive, what a waste of an immensely valuable human being!

But in his assessment of Gerald's character the chairman of the company had made a great mistake: Gerald as an enemy is pretty deadly and it was not too long before he whispered a few words into the ears of just the right person in the City. That old boys' network is pretty active still.

However, in spreading the word Gerald was not doing anything dishonourable – he simply helped to speed up a process he knew to be inevitable. A few months later the company had to call in the Receiver and the chairman lost his fat income, his Rolls and all his credibility.

Meanwhile the clouds were gathering on the domestic horizon too. Erika was demanding a divorce, quoting Gerald's transvestism as her main reason.

Gerald feared for his children: his visits to them were granted grudgingly and Erika complicated them further by creating painful scenes whenever he made his journey back to his old home, always in the hope of meeting with some measure of understanding. She greeted him with screams and violence and sent him back to me, shattered.

Outwardly Gerald took the blows philosophically. As for his dismissal, he had been expecting it, there had been rumours. He now rearranged his days to suit his new routine. Our nights got later, and so did his mornings. The house being vacant all day except for the two of us, he dressed first thing in the morning and appeared downstairs for breakfast in the most exciting apparel. I soon got used to seeing him at the breakfast table in bra, French knickers and suspender belts, sheerest nylon stockings and stiletto heels, a long gilt necklace falling over the bra, earrings dangling, as Gerry. Wearing no wig he was his most buoyantly masculine self in everything but his clothing, a sexy and easy-going Gerry, a beaming smile on his face, enjoying for the moment his new-found freedom and relief from the daily tensions at the office.

The days rolled by leisurely. He was now completely immersed in his transvestism, making the most of it, ringing several changes of clothing over the day. I had discovered a little shop with a wonderful range of fancy nighties and negligées, new but cheap, and Gerald suggested that we go there to do some shopping together, to buy garments we could both own and wear jointly. What fun! Although he was quite a bit taller than me, our measurements were the same, now that I had slimmed myself down: we both wore size 14 and a size 36B bra.

The little Welsh woman in the shop was smiling and welcoming; she saw nothing unusual in Gerald's obvious enthusiasm as he rummaged to his heart's content among the frilly see-through garments in their various hues of pinks and creams and blues and purples. His eyes lingered on a dolly nightie in brilliant turquoise – that was a must! As a contrast a long apricot-coloured see-through negligée with nightie to match followed next and two more sleeveless nightgowns delicately flowered in pink and lilac completed our purchase for the day. The little Welsh woman, still smiling, wrapped up everything and we carried our haul back home in triumph.

Surveying our wardrobe we had every reason to feel pleased: Gerald's garments mingled happily with mine, a cheerful and colourful array of dresses, skirts and blouses, evening outfits and negligées, plus quite a considerable selection of elegant shoes, belts and scarves.

Gerry looked stunning in the turquoise nightie, his handsome dark features highlighted by the contrast; his legs showed off to perfection in various fancy-coloured stockings and suspender belts. He now dreamed of getting more sets of lingerie, perhaps a Janet Reger? The prospects looked exciting . . .

However, the effects on Gerald of his various calamities had only been delayed. Simmering slowly but surely through his system, the hour came when they hit him full-force. With such force indeed that even his escape into transvestism could no longer ward it off.

And now began a strange process. Geraldine, showing no outward signs of life, though inwardly a broiling cauldron of emotions, withdrew into herself completely; she became rigid and scarcely mobile. I named the process 'cocooning'.

It was the other extreme of the lively and fun-loving Gerald, of the flamboyant and sexy Geraldine, of the exotic Gerry I knew – a quiet, introvert, utterly passive Geraldine, turned inward, numb, dumb, immobile, on her face an enigmatic little smile born of pain, reminding me of that of the Cheshire Cat in *Alice in Wonderland*.

For days on end she existed like this and I had no way of communicating with her other than administering food and drink, cigarettes, providing a chair and perhaps a cushion for her basic physical comforts. Feeling inadequate and helpless I watched her in her rigid state: immune from the outside world, immune even from me, self-contained and barely ticking over, she reminded me of a television play I had once watched of living humans being stored away in a state of deep-freeze. It chilled me.

When Geraldine cocooned it was also a test for me. Having survived my own hellfires I had for some time past felt ready to move mountains, and had proudly proclaimed this fact to anyone willing to listen. Gerald turned out to be my mountain. If I could infuse this man with some of my own new-found strength, then all my own sufferings and tribulations had been worthwhile. A strong sense of purpose took hold of me.

The days and nights of interminable and silent agony dragged on, endlessly, with no outward changes visible in Geraldine. There she sat in her corner of the black settee or on the veranda if the sun shone, motionless and with her little pathetic smile frozen on her face, her whole being prostrate and hanging in the balance, saying nothing, wanting nothing, and I felt powerless, praying that time would be her healer.

Then one morning Gerald came down, radiant. It was all over.

He was now avid for life. Appearing first thing in the morning in his most colourful and alluringly sexy apparel, breakfasting at my rustic table wearing next to nothing, adorned with plenty of jewellery, scanty bikini pants enhancing his firm and slender thighs, he introduced a strong element of fantasy into our surroundings and everything we did, until I had the greatest difficulty in distinguishing what was real and what was not.

On these occasions he rarely wore a wig; he was Gerry, the androgynous.

A few days later Gerald breathlessly announced a discovery: he had found a shop where he could hire for a nominal fee any outfit he liked from a choice of hundreds – the combinations were endless! They were theatrical costumes, meticulously authentic, and Gerald could think of little else for the moment, dreaming of all the many possibilities.

Excitedly one morning he took himself off to sift through the wealth of historic, romantic, tragic and bizarre costumes, trying on first one, then the other, having a splendid time, until he found the one that was the absolute match for his current mood of exhibitionism and flamboyance: it was a Spanish costume, bright red and sleeveless, the bodice overlaid with plenty of black lace; three flouncy tiers, richly gathered and in the same brilliant red, fell from the waist down to the ankles and opened up in front almost to the navel. A tall black mantilla of matching lace was to sit on the head, cascading down to well beneath the shoulders and almost down to the waist, the top crowned by a rose of the brightest scarlet. The costume had a name: 'Carmen Miranda'.

Gerald was brimming over with excitement: he could not wait to become Carmen Miranda and to show himself off in front of an admiring public. He made his preparations with meticulous care. He journeyed to Barkers of Kensington to have his wig dressed by Larry. Back home he applied extra strong make-up to match the brightly coloured costume. The fingernails were glued into place. His best black stockings, sheer and seamed, and the 4 inch stiletto heeled shoes showed off his well-shaped legs to perfection when glimpsed through the front opening of the costume.

All this together with her dark gypsy features made Carmen Miranda look the authentic Spanish seductress . . . she was now ready, and truly, she looked stunning!

Applying the last touches to herself in the large mirror she could not wait to be seen and admired.

We rushed off to the Pembrook to celebrate her costume. She made a remarkable entrance to surprised looks even in this haven of the unconventional. Several of the 'ladies' present were themselves wearing unusual and eye-catching outfits, but Carmen Miranda topped the lot.

The atmosphere that night was wonderful. The music blared out loud, the lights never stopped flashing, the multiple characters mixed and mingled, danced, drank and flirted, to make new friends, to meet partners for a night of sex, the outgoing, the shy, the adventurers and the frustrated, all in a melting pot here tonight, forgetting for the moment the loneliness that awaited them later.

Carmen Miranda was radiant, knowing herself to be the highlight of the evening, needing to be the centre of attention. The astonished and admiring looks she got were a balm to her hungry ego. Valerie of the slender body and the beautiful hair came over and seated herself at the table with us, looked intently at Carmen Miranda and asked straight out, 'Is *this* how you feel?'

Swiftly, like the flutter of a bird's wing and barely visible, a look of resignation fleeted over the features of Carmen Miranda, and was gone, but there was no reply.

I had the feeling that Valerie understood a very great deal, having herself been through the mill.

The evening was a great success, and we stayed until late into the night, Carmen Miranda soaking herself to bursting point with all the attention she continued to attract.

Back home in the early hours we filled our glasses, turned on the music, lit the bedroom candle, and I laid myself by Carmen Miranda, joined my mouth to hers, embracing both her body and her grief, and loved her, loved her . . .

Making our way home the following weekend we noticed a group of policemen patrolling the road, when one of them stepped forward to stop a car in front. Geraldine froze for a brief moment, then drove past the scene slowly with all the outward signs of apparent calm.

But the incident had triggered off latent fears in Gerald. It was in the early hours of the morning that I was woken by a movement, by sound, by light – Gerald was sitting straight upright in bed, pale and shaking.

I know about nightmares. Ogres and witches, demons and bitches, gargoyles, sadists and cruel foes; leering and jeering, hounding and pounding. I know. I smoothed Gerald's forehead gently, trying to bring him back to us, to me, to our own cosy little world. 'It is only a dream after all, just a dream, nothing more, shush!'

But the nightmare was not that easily got rid of. 'Let us talk about it, Gerald, let us share it, let us tear it to pieces and render it impotent. Let us kill it. Shall we laugh at it?'

This had been Gerald's dream:

A dark road, deserted and eerily silent; only Geraldine who sits huddled in her car. A sudden noise, and two heads appear at the window, two policemen larger than life demand to see her licence. Geraldine starts fumbling for it when the bigger of the two men digs his hand into her bag and pulls it out. Reads GERALD TILSON printed in large black letters. The policeman lowers his face close to Geraldine's, stares hard and drags her out of the car, then runs his paws all over her body, groping, laughing, jeering . . .

Suffocating with shame and fear Gerald had woken. I hurriedly put on a tape of our most soothing music, then quickly made Gerald a cup of tea, hot and steaming, to disperse those menacing ghosts – if I could. Sadly I realised that those ghosts may remain with Gerald always, that with all the best will in the world I might not be able to banish them forever.

A few days later we invited Marilyn to dinner. We had discovered her at the Pembrook. Dear Marilyn, blonde and lively, warm as a newly baked loaf and earthy as a young summer's day, she was a transsexual waiting for her operation. In her past she had been Mark, a husband, had grown side whiskers, had trained as a fireman, all in order to convince herself of her true masculinity, but in vain. After years of struggle she had finally had to face up to the truth, and now she had been on female hormones for over a year. Her breasts were her own and so was her full head of blonde and curly hair. Some of her facial hair had already been removed, and now there was only one more major obstacle in the way. She dressed simply and tastefully with a flair for the elegant, choosing quiet shades to suit her pale and gold complexion. Her speech was emphasized by vivid gestures of her white, soft and feminine hands, her arms were beautifully rounded and quite smooth.

Geraldine, finding herself in such congenial company and able to let her hair down, virtually, got carried away. She revelled in her role as hostess, having cooked us a superb meal, *coq-au-vin*, a great speciality of hers, and topped this up with champagne. Feeling wonderfully at ease the 'mood' came over her, she sparkled and shone, quite literally, as she had sprayed herself with glitter for the occasion, her black velvet dress – mine – flattering her hair, face and figure. Relentlessly she drew both of us right into her bewitching and magical circle, casting a spell of impish cheekiness and make-belief over Marilyn and myself, turning on her most irresistible and seductive charms, making our heads reel until we both felt dizzy and intoxicated, intoxicated with Geraldine, our faces flushed and feverish.

As the night progressed a feeling of recklessness came over Geraldine and the sleeveless white dress with the flouncy collar, the one she had worn on our special and memorable day in the storm, went to a delighted Marilyn in one of Geraldine's moments of impulsive generosity.

Alas, Marilyn felt herself becoming increasingly drawn to Gerald when she met him again a few days later, dressed in ancient jeans and an old brown pullover, much in contrast to the Carmen Miranda she had met only a few weeks before. To Gerald, however, she was not a girl, and the picture I took of them both that day showed Marilyn gently holding on to Gerald's arm and leaning against him, smiling, with Gerald backing away from her with an expression of wide-eyed alarm.

When, much later, Marilyn asked Gerald if he would consider her as a female, he was quite clear, 'Not pre-op, no, but post-op, yes!'

It was three o'clock in the morning; I was sitting up in bed where I had been waiting up all night for Gerald, who had gone to meet Erika to discuss details of their forthcoming divorce.

He entered, slim and dapper, wearing his dark blue Pierre Cardin suit, white shirt and blue tie, his teeth brilliant in his handsome face as he smiled to greet me. He took my breath away. I loved him, I loved him!

Seating himself beside me on the bed, his voice soft and controlled, he gave me all the facts: the house which was once their home was to be put on the market, the contents were to be split up, disposed of; the children . . .

Studying his face closely I could see the relief and the pain, both. Relief because matters had at long last been aired and were out in the open, pain because of the loss of his family. The date for the fatal day had been fixed, and now there was no going back.

I could not bear to see Gerald leave for his little room upstairs, to be all alone with his guilt and his pain, and so I made up a second bed on the floor next to my pine bed, to be near him, to provide human warmth and companionship, to fend off his loneliness. To my surprise Gerald was overwhelmed at this, tears springing into his eyes. How deprived of love in its true sense he must have been to be so moved by my simple gesture?

There was little else I could do for him. Gerald would have to fight his terrors all alone.

And just as I had feared, after all his beautiful relaxing there were signs that Gerald was once again about to cocoon.

There was no way whatever in which I could ward this off. Inevitably and with brutal force the pain invaded Gerald, gnawed at his inside and took over completely, showing no mercy, no slacking, no let-up.

The painfully silent nights and days followed one another interminably and time once again lost all meaning. No words, no music, no relief of any kind. I was tempted to touch this silence, rip it open and let in sound. All the uproar was inside Geraldine, who was now once more sitting huddled in her corner of the settee, motionless.

And then, just as on that last time, the grieving over, Gerald emerged once more eager to devour life, greedy for it.

Some time ago Gerald had discovered a three-piece outfit consisting of negligée and two nightdresses, colourful, sleek and elegant, see-through, sexy and revealing. Full of frills and gatherings, they were a transvestite's dream. He had found this treasure tucked away in the back room of a secondhand shop in Fulham, waiting to be rescued.

Being out of work did not equip Gerald with lots of funds, and so he had to wait awhile, trying his self-restraint and patience not a little. Now at last the day had come when he had the necessary means and so off we both went for the great purchase. Gerald was already known to the woman in charge, who greeted me as his 'good lady' – did she perhaps take me for Gerald's wife? If so, it was flattering. My darling beautiful boy – how proud I was to be with him!

The ensemble was a riot of colours. Hanging there in the obscurity of the dim little back room, squeezed in among inferior and much less splendid companions, hidden between piles of shabby cast-offs and old hats, it seemed quite out of place.

It was made of such thin material, it was so smooth to the touch it seemed almost liquid. Gerald's face, while removing these delicate garments from their hiding place, assumed an expression of ecstasy, his eyes shining as he handed them to the lady for payment.

That night, when wearing these flowing robes, Gerry looked like a large exotic bird, in suspender belts and stockings and high-heeled shoes, about to be airborne, mysterious and secretive, his facial expression and demeanour in complete harmony with the garments he wore. It was as if these frilly pieces of ultra-feminine clothing inspired Gerry, as if they were capable of imbuing him with their innermost meaning, hidden from the rest of us.

The night was mellow. We stood facing one another in the middle of the room, the warm balmy air and the scent from the garden overflowing through the open door of the veranda and we listened to the soft music – was it Rodrigo's Guitar Concerto? The air was still, there was nothing and nobody in the whole world, only Gerry and the music, and I.

And as the swelling waves of the sounds filled the space around us, gently at first and in perfect unison with it, Gerry's body began to sway, moving rhythmically from side to side like that of a belly dancer, slowly, languorously at first, becoming ever faster and more ecstatic, until the sounds of the waves reached a resounding crescendo and carried us both away into a perfect trance.

'My Bird of Paradise in your colourful plumage, my songbird, my mysterious and exotic lover, you who bring all the riches of my dreams into my life, how can I bear so much mystery, so much beauty?' I felt weak and my legs began to give way, so that I had to lie down, just stopping myself from falling.

Half reclining on the bed I watched enthralled as Gerry moved sensuously to the sounds. His eyes had a life of their own tonight, they had their feverish look. My bedroom was no longer the room I knew so well, it was transformed into a magic circle, the atmosphere unreal, myself bewitched by my sorcerer...

Stretched out on the bed before him I gently reached out with one leg to touch his thigh where it showed bare above the stocking as he danced to the music, and Gerry responded at once as if electrified by that touch; we were both under a spell as the movements of the figure before me became ever more ecstatic, beautiful, yet strangely bizarre.

Truly, he was my Bird of Paradise.

God help me, how I loved his contrasts, his versatility! I had always been intrigued by opposites. It seemed to me that without good and evil, happiness and pain, light and shade, there could be no conflict, no struggle, no growth, no life. Gerald, like some Eastern deity being male and female all in one was a microcosm all his own, but being so privileged he had to pay the worldly price: being misunderstood, jeered at, at best tolerated. It had forced him to go through life wearing a mask.

You may ask: what is it like to make love to a man who not only dresses as a woman, but who tries to move as a woman, think as a woman, feel like one? A man who enjoys making love in sexy lingerie and who expects his partner to be dressed likewise?

Do not forget that I was in love! In love with a man

who was different, who was special, a man who was in conflict with himself, wanting desperately to conform but unable to do so, a man whose suffering was acute because he could not keep to those standards which his whole upbringing had taught him to regard as the only correct and desirable ones. The fact that he felt guilty and despised himself for not being able to toe the line aroused in me a strong feeling of compassion, of pity even, and all my maternal feelings took over. He was my darling man, my lover, he was also the child whom I needed to protect from suffering and surround with love, helping him to become strong and resilient.

My love of adventure and of colour did the rest. Gerald was exciting! Exciting beyond all words. In Geraldine all my senses found fulfillment. In my drab past these senses had withered away, starved of nourishment, but now I could sate them all: my sense of smell with the waft of our special scent, my ears with our soft romantic music, my taste buds with Gerald's imaginative cooking, my sense of touch with the touching of Geraldine or Gerry, and as for my eyes, they had a veritable feast: from the stark beauty of Gerald's nakedness right through to all the stages of an elaborately dressed Geraldine – a feast of shape, of colour, of texture.

Suddenly, here was all the colour that I had ever craved for in all my life, all the colours of the rainbow, a whole riot of it; suddenly here was an abundance, right there in the privacy of my own home, for me to revel in. I had been so hungry for it all, the more I partook the more I wanted. Oh yes – I was going to revel – I was going to revel all I could!

And he had liberated my sex, had opened up to me that chapter which for so long had been so firmly closed to me.

As Gerald he had introduced me to a whole new vocabulary, always with the greatest care, never rushing me. In my old world these words had been forbidden and were never mentioned, and I had not known the meaning of them. Suddenly they sprang to life, Gerald in his alter-ego rejoicing in his wonderful body, loving his sex, needing to give as much as take. Whether in his role as Geraldine or as Gerry, Gerald most of the time acted just as any other lusty male, though never a macho one. Always sensitive and deeply aware of me, with a marvellous intuition, he liberated sex for me, made me blossom out, giving me at this late stage my first spring ever.

Did I ever feel I was making love to a woman? No way! Though I pretended often and enjoyed it. Enjoyed it because Geraldine thrilled to it, and I was greedy for her, wanted the whole of her; by having the whole of Geraldine I was having the whole of Gerald, all barriers removed.

Stroking Geraldine's breasts was enjoyable to me, because to her it was the ultimate proof that she was a woman – at that moment. Who am I to go into the ins and outs of such a nature? If she was thrilled and excited, so was I! We breathed and loved as one. Sometimes, when Geraldine and I were wonderfully entwined I would remove my mouth from hers and say, 'How I wish that His Grey Eminence could see us now!' And we would kill ourselves with laughter at the preposterous thought of it.

VI

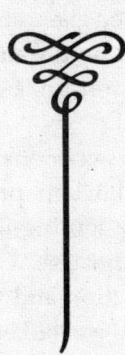

Tonight we had guests for dinner. Alan was a transvestite, a friend from the Pembrook, and he brought with him his wife Margaret. Margaret was a pleasant little woman, round and wholesome as a dumpling, chatty and maternal, and she and I hit it off at once by talking about our families.

Margaret and Alan had been married for nineteen years before Alan had let his wife into his secret. Until then he had successfully hidden his alter-ego by cross-dressing inside the family car. He had not told Margaret until he felt the marriage was strong enough to carry the blow and survive. It did, but Margaret had not found it easy to come to terms with her husband's strange habit of turning himself into a female at regular intervals.

On arrival at our house Alan quickly disappeared

into the bedroom to change in comfort and a few minutes later re-emerged as Ann. Ann turned out to be very plain – a female with specs and straight hair, plain skirt and blouse all in greys and blacks, miles removed from Geraldine with her glamour and allure, sparkling with glitter tonight. I saw Geraldine eyeing Ann with disapproval, but Margaret put her hand on Ann's arm reassuringly: all is well.

As always on these occasions Geraldine had spent the afternoon in the kitchen producing a wonderful meal and she was now serving it up, a task she loved: she made the perfect hostess. Candles and music set everything off to perfection and the drink did the rest: tongues loosened and we talked, completely at ease with one another. I watched Geraldine with fascination as she slowly drifted into her mood of rascality, become more and more animated and carried away by the minute. Anything is likely to happen with Geraldine in this excited state, sooner or later she was sure to lead on to her favourite topic of sex and talk about it in the frankest way: 'Mona and I made love this afternoon – it was *fabulous*!' she exclaimed, her eyes sparkling with fun and impishness as she went on to recount her most recent memories . . .

She looked ravishing tonight. She wore a simple black dress, tight fitting and adorned only by a gold necklace and earrings to match, a gilt bracelet emphasizing her lovely arms. Her slim waist showed up to advantage and so did her shapely long legs. She was a perfect beauty.

The meal over and having got to know one another a little better, Geraldine was unable to contain herself any longer. She begged Ann to follow her into the bedroom; she was absolutely dying to improve Ann's appearance.

And now Geraldine the perfectionist came into her own. She used all her considerable skill with make-up on the lucky Ann, she took off her own wig and put it on Ann's head, thus endowing her with her own dark curls. She insisted that Ann take off her blouse and skirt and replace them with an elegant twenties dress in heavy satin of the deepest royal blue, sleeveless and with a very low plunge at the back centering in a large bow, heavy drapes gathering across front and neck. Lastly, she removed Ann's glasses.

As Ann re-emerged from the bedroom she looked stunningly transformed. Her legs now exposed to well above the knees and conscious of her elegant dress, she moved very much more gracefully and quite differently from the Ann of half an hour ago. Her hands and bare arms had acquired a more elaborate and lively way of gesturing, and her face in the new wig and minus the glasses was subtly changed. Geraldine stood back and admired her handiwork with pleasure: she had created an attractive female where before there had been a sexless spinster.

But Margaret looked at Ann uneasily; she did not know what to make of it all. If this were just play-acting she could have laughed it off, but alas, it was not play-acting, and she knew it. This was a part of her husband she had not come across until tonight, and before long her eyes were filling with tears.

Seeing the little woman in distress, Geraldine's heart

melted with remorse; she could not have foreseen such a reaction, it was all meant to be such good fun. She decided to undo the damage. Simply overflowing with compassion she commenced to pay Margaret all the compliments at her disposal, praising her pretty little face, the lovely eyelashes, going into every detail the way only a lover should – intimate and flattering, making her feel important and beautiful, pampered and feminine, until Margaret revived and slowly began to glow. Geraldine was now in her element, a natural at this, and within moments she had Margaret in the bedroom too, not to make love to I hasten to add, but to transform her as well, to make her up beautifully, dress her in my wig (the one I could never bring myself to wear) and to spray her abundantly with scent and glitter.

When Margaret re-entered the dining room she, too, was transformed and quite an equal to her husband in glamour.

But Geraldine had not finished yet. For her the most important part of the evening was still to come, the moment she had been planning and waiting for. Choosing a time when everyone was cheerfully relaxed and with wine and conversation flowing, she popped The Question. She addressed herself to Margaret directly: 'Do you allow Alan to make love to you as Ann?' is what she needed to know.

The answer was all-important – it was part of Gerald's search for a new future. Leaving me out for the moment, he wanted to know: is it possible to combine Gerald and Geraldine with married life to a 'normal' woman?

But Margaret looked confused. All her cheer evaporated very quickly and this time she absolutely could not contain herself any longer: she burst into a flood of tears and sobbed her little heart out, desperately.

She discarded her wig with double-speed and tried to become her old self once more, back to normal. Geraldine tried to smooth things over again, but matters had gone too far this time, and in any case the hour was late.

Alan and Margaret took their leave.

It had been a most eventful dinner party.

It must have been nearing 3 o'clock in the morning, and the impish Geraldine who had ruled over our evening was now making love to me. She had taken off her black velvet dress and was wearing only her silken petticoat over girdle and stockings, though she had kicked off the shiny sling-backs on to the floor below. I had eased off her frilly French knickers and they, too, lay on the floor. As for me, I was equally encased in cami-knickers of the palest apricot over my black corselette and was wearing my sheerest seamed stockings.

Geraldine reached out to turn on the tape recorder where it stood on the small table by the bedside, next to two unfinished tumblers of wine. Her heady scent made me giddy. From the other side of the room the red candle in the large glass jar sent over a warm, flickering light, illuminating Geraldine's face, her black eyes laughing down at me, cheeky, playful, teasing . . .

This was now our new pattern: Gerald had thrown his lot in with his brother, helping him to run the family business; three days of each week away from me, four days, five nights, dedicated to us!

With Gerald gone the house was dead. My familiar surroundings had lost their charm, their meaning, they were black, bleak and dull, and so were our sexy clothes, the silken underwear wasting away in the drawers, the elegant dresses and nighties hanging uselessly in the wardrobe. This house which I had loved only moments before now yawned at me, silent like a graveyard; in it I moved like a mechanical doll.

I grabbed the telephone like a life-saver, urgently dialling Louisa's number: I needed to talk about Gerald, to infuse some glimmering of life into my dead hours.

How many seconds in a minute? How many in an hour, in a day? And how many in a night?

Then, one morning I woke, my body tingling: he would be back tonight! Soon after midday I started to lay out the clothes for Geraldine, arranging each garment lovingly on the bed to show it off to its best advantage, her dress for tonight, the night of her return to me. I knew that she would long for a tight corselette after her absence, and for something soft and feminine to go on top.

Quite soon my lover was to be with me! My ears did not miss the sound of a single car or of footsteps approaching, my heart threatened to jump out of its confined space each time a door slammed shut. Occasionally Gerald was late and I had listened to so many car doors being slammed that I was tense and drained long before he arrived.

He had come – I recognised the way he turned the key in its lock, the exact way the door clicked to when he closed it behind him, I knew the sound of the few steps he took before opening the door of the room where I stood waiting for him. He was even more striking than I had remembered – he was back, my incredible lover! He greeted me, beaming, his dark eyes simply dancing in his head, and although all he said was 'Hi, Mona,' I felt flushed and intoxicated and as I looked at all the familiar objects around me I found they were once more imbued with magic and quite definitely not of this world.

From time to time Geraldine would feel the need to be a young maiden, and dream of being seduced, and dress all in white.

'My snow-white darling, you who are so pure and virginal, I love you. I love your eyes – let me kiss them – I love your lips – open them and let me taste them, let me caress your neck, your shoulders, your breasts – I worship you. Do not fear that I may hurt you, my darling. I would sooner endure torture myself than injure one hair of your body, trust me. I will love and shield you from all evil, you who are so pure and as clear as the waters streaming from the mountain tops.'

As we became ever closer Gerald's frustration at our age gap grew. We were so perfectly atuned to one another, we both would have chosen to remain together and we would have loved to have children. Gerald adores children, he dreams of family life, of hearing the patter of little feet around him, and this is something I could not do for him. In our so beautiful and perfect relationship there had been from the very beginning a strong element of tragedy, the knowledge that one day . . . after all, I was the exact age of his own mother! If I cried over the fact that I was unable to carry his child, for him this was quite equally frustrating.

'It is a tragedy that you are not younger!' he stormed into the room. The cursing and raging did not help. Cold facts and figures were staring us in the face, and somehow we had to come to terms with them.

'Do you mind me fantasising, Mona? Does it hurt you? Well then! Supposing you were younger and we were married. I would work so hard for you, and we would have children, and you would lack nothing.

'Then, one day, I would have come home and said,

"Mona, I've seen a fantastic house, come and look at it." And you'd say, "Oh, but I am very happy here – I don't want to move to another house." And then I would say, "Ah – but wait till you see this one!" And you'd come and look at it, and say, "Oh – YES!" '

The day of the divorce over, Gerald announced that a double-bed would arrive shortly, to replace the narrow pine bed which had had to serve as our love bed until now. 'I will show you what a *real* marriage can be like. From now on, Mona, you will have a part-time, live-in husband.'

This time I did not object. On the contrary, I rejoiced! I no longer feared the loss of my independence or that we might destroy something precious and wonderful by living together; I was now confident that the closer we could get the more beautiful our relationship would become and that, together, we would go from strength to strength.

Soon afterwards a large double-bed was delivered to my house, and Gerald moved in with his landlady. Geraldine had long made use of my wardrobe downstairs, now Gerald's suits, shirts and trousers moved in too, making themselves at home, to my utmost delight.

Quite apart from anything else, I found living with this transvestite enormously exciting and stimulating, his fetishism adding a magic and charm to everything he did. There was not the slightest chance of my ever being overcome with boredom, a bugbear which had bedevilled me with almost every other man in the past. If I left the house I never knew who would await me on my return: Gerald, Geraldine, or Gerry? I was in love with all of them! The variations and in-between shades were infinite, not only of dress, but also of character.

In Gerald I had a charming friend, completely masculine in every gesture, thought and action. If he was not my lover, I was fully compensated by the warm camaraderie which had grown up between us. He was forceful and decisive yet always helpful and considerate; we needed to be close to one another in all the giving and taking of everyday life, loving the companionship and domesticity. He was also a wizard about the house, and could repair my hi-fi, fix a broken lock and get the fireplace into working order, all in a morning before changing into one of his alter-egos.

Watching Gerald the handyman change from worn-out jeans and shirt into the colourful array of Gerry or Geraldine and in doing so become quite another kind of person was an exhilarating experience each time, not to be missed, an experience of incredulity and wonder, exciting and enriching. Gerald quite simply had the gift to interpret his moods and feelings through the choice of his garments. Others write poetry, make pots, act or express themselves in music or painting. Gerald found complete satisfaction in expressing himself in the way he dressed, and he preferred to do so in female clothing.

Like all true transvestites Gerald worshipped women. He studied them endlessly in order to perfect his *femme* side, he was constantly observing and learning. Though I sometimes thought that he by-passed the many modern young women who had happily discarded make-up, long hair, high heels and often even a skirt. Something in him seemed to have fixed the female image invariably with long hair and lashes, pretty face and with immaculate make-up, soft lingerie and high-heeled shoes.

The fact that Gerald adored women and tried to be one from time to time, also meant that he was able to put himself into my frame of mind when making love to me as Geraldine. In that state he knew with an uncanny perception my innermost feelings, my likes and my hatreds, my every reaction. In making love he aimed at the highest peaks, the creation of the fantasy being a vital part of our foreplay, with sensitivity, consideration and a romantic setting being a natural part of the scene. I do not believe that it would have been possible for him to hurt a woman or slight her feelings while he was Geraldine.

Though Gerald the male could hurt, and to judge from my limited experience of him was a pretty clumsy lover too. I can only suppose that in this state he neither possessed the facility nor the desire to put himself into his partner's frame of mind and understand her every whim. And when in a state of guilt he could deride with the best of them. In the beginning his remarks had been aimed at our age gap, or simply at the fact that I was not Erika. I had persevered because this man had fascinated and intrigued me, and I had become far too deeply involved to let go. Later, as our relationship developed beyond anything we could have foreseen, the remarks were never to be repeated.

How could I ever forget those words that Gerry said

to me one night by the flicker of the bedroom candle – and remember that Gerry was half Gerald and half Geraldine: 'To me you are ageless – you are just Mona. I love you!'

Gerald was under a heavy cloud, in danger of being crushed by his compassion, by his love for his fellow-creatures, for old friends from his childhood, for people who loved him in return because he knew how to respect them, how to encourage them to give of their best, to cooperate with him on every level.

Circumstances had forced Gerald to dismiss a number of people who had worked for his brother's company for many years, who had given their all and had helped to make it a success in better times before the depression had set in, people who had almost become part of the family. Gerald had called them all together to explain the situation carefully, showing them that he had no alternative if the company was to survive. And the company meant work for the lucky ones who could carry on.

He returned from this ordeal, tears in eyes and voice, and for the next few days showed signs of renewed cocooning. Every single individual, every family who had been put out of work because of his decision, weighed on his conscience like a mammoth boulder. He had been forced into doing the rational thing, and it was he who had had to make the final selection, playing God.

How to dissolve that dilemma? My warm, my compassionate Gerald, I loved him for his compassion for his fellow men as much as I loved him for the love he bore his children.

There was only one way out for him. Soon there followed the escape into his fantasy, the reality being much too horrible to contemplate.

And yet he could be very ruthless. When it came to beating a competitor in business he had no qualms whatsoever. Those were the rules of the game, and anyone entering that game must be prepared to be beaten into pulp, and he had no misgivings whatever in doing all the pulping with his own two hands. On the contrary, he thrived on this kind of fight, enjoyed coming out of it victorious, feeling that he had achieved something worthwhile. And if by any chance he was the loser – well, he had played the game to the best of his ability, and he had been unlucky. But he would sure make a come-back!

When it came to the fight of men among men, Gerald was a born winner.

Marilyn, our transsexual friend from the Pembrook, had at long last had her operation. I took myself off to visit her, flowers from me in one hand, a bottle of Marilyn's favourite scent from an absent Gerald in the other.

Marilyn's head was resting against the white pillows, her face almost as white. She had braved this excruciating operation without ever a doubt in her mind that it was the only thing to do, because of her need to become as complete a woman as medical science will allow her. Her body might feel frail for the moment, but her spirit was undaunted and she was happy that it was all over at long last, this operation towards which she had striven, worked and saved up for so many years. The most painful stage, though, was still to come: several months of dilating her new vagina. Marilyn was going to withstand it because she had one all-consuming wish: to be able to live and work as a normal woman. She dreamt of love and romance with a nice macho man, having been driven into the fringe world for far too many years, ever since Mark had decided to face the truth about himself and live life as Marilyn. Society had pushed Marilyn into that fringe world, and now she could not wait to leave it; she hoped to get married one day and adopt children, whom she adored. Even as things stood now, though, she would not be able to get married with the blessings of either State or Church in this, her own country. Her birth certificate described her as male. I felt full of admiration for the Marilyns of this world, be they transsexual or anything else, they have the courage to face up to themselves and to overcome every obstacle put in their way.

Gerald wrote: 'All my love, Marilyn, and I do hope that you will withstand the pain of the operation and rise to full womanhood to stand alongside your sisters. Just think of the advantages you will have over the other women!

'May you find all the happiness you deserve, Marilyn. With our deepest love and admiration, from Mona and Gerald/ine.'

VII

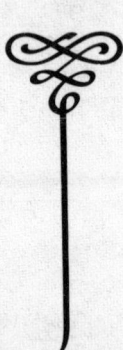

Christmas was in the air – what to give my lover-mistress, my part-time husband? I had often observed Gerald leafing through the glossy women's magazines, greedily eyeing the more luxuriant adverts of ladies' underwear displayed in their pages – I took my clue from there. Janet Reger was a name new to *me*, but it appeared that to possess garments graced with her label was the ultimate in self-indulgence, and so, towards that Mecca of sexy underwear in New Bond Street I directed my steps, cheque-book at the ready.

From the wealth of colours and designs that met my eyes I chose a three-piece set consisting of bikini pants, bra and suspender belt made of the most luscious of flimsy materials in shiny pillar-box red. Lavishly laced with delicate appliqué in off-white, each piece was further embellished with a tiny cluster of red flowers and minute naughty bows. Picturing Gerald in them my heart almost missed a beat . . . they would go ideally with his dark looks, and I hoped most passionately that he would be thrilled with them.

Boxing day found me with my family in a sleepy country setting. We were assembled in the large drawing room, the green lawns from the garden almost overflowing beneath the french windows and into the house, to blend with the equally green carpets under our feet. Leisurely we had whiled away the hours with eating and playing games, eating and playing . . .

Into this peaceful setting arrived Gerald for the afternoon. Dark blue Pierre Cardin suit, white shirt dazzling at cuffs and neck, handsome almost beyond belief, he was the ultimate in worldly sophistication, contrasting strongly with our relaxed, pastel-shaded, chintzy surroundings. Making use of a moment when everyone's attention was on a game of charades, I rested my hand lightly on Gerald's back – he jerked round sharply like a coil too tightly wound, and looked at me with the eyes of Geraldine – I could see at once that he could not wait to rid himself of all his conventional male finery, to revel in a riot of femininity and erotic fantasy.

The afternoon over we raced back home, we could not wait!

It was our first chance to be alone with one another for over a whole week. Quickly I lit the fire in the grate and piled on logs, and immediately our room was transformed by the warm glow, all the decorations around us began to glitter and sparkle and the little tree in the window proudly preened itself, ablaze with countless tiny multicoloured lights. We were once more transported into our world of magic and make-belief.

The moment had come to exchange presents. Gerald handed me the small box; it contained my very first pair of earrings. He was not a bit ceremonious about it all, as if embarrassed, and I thought that he must find it difficult. I knew that he could be generous to a fault – but who, actually, was giving me the present? It was of necessity Gerald who had to do the purchasing, yet I belonged mainly to Geraldine. And Geraldine preferred to be spoiled, rather than to spoil.

Whereas I *loved* giving!

Gerald became excited as he saw the Janet Reger name printed on the flat package I handed him.

He opened it hurriedly, impatiently, and exclaimed as he saw the garments in their brilliant red colouring showing up against their background of snow-white tissue – I had chosen right!

He lost no time in ridding himself of the Pierre Cardin suit and all else, and now, one by one, slowly, savouring every moment, I eased over his lovely body the soft garments; they seemed to be created especially for him, caressing him and showing off his beauty to perfection. If only Janet Reger could have seen him – I felt sure she would have approved.

That night we christened our new presents by making love slowly – slowly and sensuously, in front of the blazing log fire. I was wearing my new earrings, dressed recklessly at my most seductive, and Gerald – now in Geraldine's curls – wore nothing but his new lingerie, his body aglow.

We were so lucky! How many lovers were there, I wondered to myself, able to let go of all pretence and inhibitions, waive all spectre of prejudice, of caution, and yet merge ever closer into one another? I had submerged myself so much into Gerald, the time came when I began to feel that I *was* him! Perhaps this was a necessity, Gerald being so enigmatic, incorporating so many alter-egos. There was no way at all in which I could have understood this man from the outside.

Nor could I have submerged myself to such an extent if Gerald had not been so eminently loveable, so affectionate, so witty and charming, such a challenging and exciting lover, so unrestrainedly sexy and such a great friend. There was no reason at all why I should withhold any of myself, why I should not become wholly him.

It was a state of bliss. By becoming Gerald and yet in a strange and important way retaining my Monica personality, I likened myself to people I had heard claim were able to detach their souls from their bodies, observing their own physical actions from a distance.

Watching Gerald grow with confidence I was filled with an unspeakable happiness, with joy. Yet I knew full well that a confident and healthy Gerald would of necessity need to go farther afield, to seek his future elsewhere and away from me. And therefore my happiness was amply interlaced with pain. Having absorbed his being into mine, I could no longer visualise life without him.

VIII

Every true transvestite dreams of the great day when he finally dares to face the world at large as a female, and the world accepts him, asking no questions.

If 'she' gets 'read' she dies a thousand deaths, but if she passes, her happiness is unequalled.

Gerald was no exception to this dream.

His time had come.

For the sake of caution we had decided on the nearby park for Geraldine's first outing.

Dressing herself as sensibly as she knew how and borrowing my fur coat for the occasion, Geraldine took an eternity over her make-up. If she was to reveal her features in the harsh daylight she would need the most meticulous preparation and a whole new technique of concealment, a daunting task.

The afternoon was bright and sunny as we left the house for the car standing on the corner. Would Geraldine go down as genuine? Or would we bump into a friend or neighbour who would recognise Geraldine as Gerald in wig and woman's dress? The thought was too horrific to contemplate! Pretending a calm we did not feel we managed to get into the car, unrecognised, safe for the moment.

On reaching the park we made for the least populated areas, Geraldine stalking the soft ground in her 4 inch heels. From time to time a few people would stroll past us, unsuspecting, sometimes smiling a 'good afternoon'. It reassured us. I heaved a sigh of relief each time I saw they were strangers: I know a great many people in my neighbourhood. In the case of a chance encounter, how exactly was I to introduce Geraldine?

However, we were lucky. We did not walk for long, Geraldine as eager as I was to get back home to safety. We had accomplished an important 'first'.

It was the beginning of Geraldine's liberation, and the beginning of a new person altogether.

It was the birth of Dina.

Dina was by no means born overnight. The process of her gestation was comparatively short and lasted for just a few weeks. Her birth was slow, painful, and quite inexplicable. How do I describe the inexplicable? I'll try!

God only knows that by living with the Gerald-Geraldine-Gerry combination I had had to change my ideas on a great many things, had learned to live with a man whose psyche was so complex as to defy psychologist and hypnotist alike, as well as any attempt on my part for a logical explanation; but all that had gone on before had been as nothing compared to the miracle that both Gerald and I now witnessed together.

Yes, Gerald too. What was now happening inside him was something separate from himself and quite beyond his own control. He could only watch from the outside, passively, having no say in the matter whatsoever.

Geraldine had begun to cocoon again – but with a difference. Whereas earlier she had cocooned because of pain due to the breakdown of Gerald's life as he had known it up till then, this time her cocooning had a broody aspect about it. Something new and vital was shaping and growing inside her, trying to come to the fore and force itself out of her.

The new force struggling to be free was Dina.

Her birth was tortured and difficult, the dark forces of destruction fighting to hinder the liberation of what lay within, while I had to watch the struggle helplessly from the outside, quite unable to relieve the agony. Trying to comprehend what was going on inside her I asked Geraldine for a explanation, but she only shook her head in resignation, 'I have no idea, no idea at all!' was all she was able to comment.

What earlier had been a resigned and mysterious smile and had reminded me of the Cheshire Cat had now turned into a mask of pain, Geraldine's face impenetrable.

The separation of Dina from Geraldine was uncanny, unfathomable. In my mind's eye there formed a picture of Dina emerging from Geraldine much as the butterfly emerges from its chrysalis, the process a miracle, complex and utterly mysterious, defying all rational explanation. Yet Dina was a *fait accompli*, a new and very real person who was now entering our lives and was rapidly becoming a very important part of it.

She differed profoundly from her sister, Geraldine. Dina had emerged from her chrysalis a serious and thoughtful person, unsure of herself, probing her new surroundings with caution, the way a tightrope walker might probe his rope before committing his bodyweight onto it.

She was also of necessity chaste, being new to the world, a reflective, quiet and undemonstrative young woman, so different from Geraldine the extrovert, flamboyant, glamorous and sex-loving. Dina was destined to become my platonic friend.

She was slowly taking on a new life of her own, blending smoothly with her environment, never causing so much as a flutter or a stir.

I asked Gerald how he saw Dina's future and his

face assumed a blank expression, his eyes vague. All he could do was to shrug his shoulders at me, helpless, 'I don't know, Mona, really I don't!' Which was not a bit like Gerald with his extraordinary perception, not usually lost for the right word. Though he added, 'I do not wish to stop it, I am enjoying it far too much!'

Hopeful, I now turned to Dina herself, needing to understand what was going on inside her. In vain. She shook her head slowly-slowly, her sole reply to me, her face clueless.

Dina dressed with the greatest modesty in keeping with her unassuming and pensive disposition. She was quiet and undemanding, able to sit and ponder or read for hours on end, and was slowly beginning to enjoy her new existence. Dina, the product of my relationship with Geraldine, her birthplace my home.

The appearance of Dina in our lives did not at all mean that she was to replace Geraldine or Gerry in any way. It did mean that there was yet one more person taking her place side by side with the others.

After Dina had had her fair share of appearing at home in private or on the occasional inconspicuous walk in the park, she felt the need to 'come out' fully, the next and most desirable aim being to shop for clothing. At Barkers of Kensington, of course.

Before doing so, however, Dina had to grapple with the problem of her voice. Gerald's voice, so rich and well-modulated and warmly reflecting his great emotional range was also quite definitely male, and it just would not do.

Experimenting with her voice this way and that, Dina had an inspiration: the Scottish accent lends itself well to a higher pitch, and if in addition to this she kept her voice soft, that should do it! She proposed to practise on me; she was a brilliant mimic and had no difficulty at all in reproducing the authentic Scottish accent. I listened to the unaccustomed sounds coming out of Dina's mouth and quickly stifled a giggle – but to the uninitiated, I was sure, she would sound utterly convincing.

And so, after the completion of her usual meticulous daytime preparations and wearing a simple brown pleated dress topped by my pink mac and with gloves, shoes and handbag to match, Dina and I set off in the direction of Kensington.

This was a great moment, and I had taken my camera with me to record it. The photograph in my album shows Dina walking towards me in front of the store, proudly mingling with the passers-by. Though tall and striking to look at she was in no way conspicuous and had the appearance of a most attractive and well-dressed young woman, confident and at ease with the world.

Once inside Barkers our first stop was the cosmetics counter; it had to be Orlane! Dina, just as Gerald, went only for the best – and the most expensive. Jean, who served her at the Orlane counter, 'knew', although this was the first time that she had met Dina in person. Being a good professional and discreet, she treated

Dina as befits a lady, giving her expert advice about her make-up problems. I kept myself very much in the background and watched Dina amass what seemed to me a vast selection of face creams, nail varnishes, eye-shadows, mascara.

Our next goal was the fashion department. Dina revelled in the array of dresses, skirts and blouses, and chose for herself a quiet, inconspicuous ensemble: a dark, tight-fitting skirt and to go with it a soft, cream-coloured blouse, such as any well-dressed girl might be wearing to the office. The sales lady was not aware of anything unusual, and I could see from the expression on Dina's face that she was highly pleased with her purchase as well as with herself.

And now it was my turn. Gerald in a fit of generosity had promised to treat me to a new dress, and Dina remembered! Confronted with the vast choice I did not know where to start. I wished that I could relax and muster some enthusiasm, but this I was unable to do. Thoroughly unaccustomed to my role of being given a treat by a man and feeling awkward and self-conscious, I was quite unable to make up my mind, casting questioning glances in the direction of Dina as I tried on each new dress. But Dina shook her head disapprovingly each time, until finally we decided to leave my treat for another day. Relieved, I made my way to the till to settle Dina's purchases, for in spite of all her painstaking preparations, Dina was as yet unable to summon up courage to talk to the salesgirl, or expose her person to close scrutiny across the counter. We were both impatient to get away, and being badly in need of refreshment, we now headed for the 'Retreat'.

On reaching the crowded cafeteria Dina chose a seat in the farthest corner where she could sit facing the wall, her head lowered over the table, eyes downcast, and she talked only in the softest whisper. Looking at her I thought that she must surely draw to herself the attention of all the people behind her, sitting there so self-consciously, so self-effacingly, so completely anonymously, so afraid.

On our way out to the car I asked Dina, 'Why do you always look down at the ground before you? Why do you not look at people in the way you normally do?'

Dina pondered for a moment. Then the answer came:

'I do not wish to attract the attention of a man, and I do not wish to attract a woman, so I avoid looking at people direct. Looking at a man I would feel like a homosexual, looking at a woman like a lesbian, and so I prefer to look at no one.'

Back in the car she rebuked me severely, 'I am not going to dress-shop with *you* again – you treat me as a man!' And with a guilty pang in the region of my heart I realised that I had done just that. And of course it was quite true that in whatever shape or mood my partner may have chosen to appear, to me, behind it all, there was always the strong knowledge of Gerald.

But for Dina this was the most terrible mistake. I should have treated her as I did Louisa, my woman friend and confidante. Though, whoever has heard of one woman treating another to a new dress? Not under ordinary circumstances, surely?

Today was Sunday, a Sunday in the company of the new, the quiet Dina. Although it was only February, the day was blue-skied and sunny, and we decided to take ourselves off to Hyde Park, to walk along the Serpentine for one of our rare outings, as Dina felt increasingly the need to air her new person and to 'pass'. With each time she mingled undetected her confidence, and her person, grew. Normally Dina did not care much for using her feet any more than Gerald did: he preferred to propel himself comfortably on four wheels rather than exert himself by walking, which he considered rather an unproductive activity.

Going for a stroll with Dina was strange. There was not a great deal we could say to one another, she had as yet little experience of life and therefore our conversation was of necessity limited, and it was almost like talking with a non-person. I could not hold her hand, either, as I loved doing with Gerald, or we would have looked like a couple of lesbians, which decidedly we were not.

As we passed by the river boats, the picnickers sitting on the grass, the riders on horseback trotting along the bridle paths, I could not help wishing that Dina would change into Geraldine, or Gerald, so that we might communicate like any other normal two people. Dina, however, smiled happily throughout our walk. For her, to blend into the lively, teeming scene around us was exactly what she needed, and no more.

On our return home she informed me that the afternoon had been 'absolutely perfect' and that she had enjoyed herself immensely.

With the evening approaching Dina asked me to fetch some of her more exotic garments. She took off the new sedate skirt and cream blouse in front of the fire, and as she did so, became more lively and free by the minute; she discarded her wig and for just one brief moment, bare of all adornments, was Gerald. I now pulled over Gerald's body the tight corselette, black lace on dark red, to be topped only by the see-through negligée in apricot, thin as cobwebs and edged with black. Panties, stockings and stilettoes perfected the ensemble, and now, wigless, before me stood Gerry as my companion for the night.

Eyes impish and full of fun, overflowing with good humour and conversation sparkling, Gerry was exhilarating company as we sat down to food and wine by the light of the candle, soft music filling the air around us, and we both of us wished that time would pass us by, forget about us and leave us alone, leave us like this forever.

Several weeks had passed, and Dina had grown considerably in stature.

We found ourselves once more at Barkers; this time Dina faced the sales ladies without hesitation and dealt with all the payments herself, too. All went splendidly, without a hitch. Or almost. Unbeknown to Dina who was utterly absorbed in choosing a dress for herself, I had noticed a young couple staring at her and whispering. I broke into a cold sweat: had Dina been 'read'? If so, she must on no account be made aware of it!

Pushing myself between Dina and the couple I gently manoeuvred her in the opposite direction, as far from them as I could. The danger passed. Perhaps they mistook her striking looks for those of a famous pop-star? You never know!

This time Dina entered the 'Retreat' with an air of gusto. Seating herself at the most prominent table right by the entrance, she openly faced the incoming public as they entered in search of refreshment. Legs stretched out long in front and easing herself comfortably back into her chair with an air of nonchalance, this self-assured young woman looked all and sundry straight in the eyes. Coffee by her side, cigarette in hand, she enjoyed herself immensely.

Dina had been liberated.

And so, too, had Gerald.

He now accepted himself as the person he was and that included Geraldine, Dina and Gerry. He could live and explore to the full each one of them in the reassuring knowledge that they were loved and accepted by me as part of his whole and exciting personality.

And now that all his guilt feelings had at long last

evaporated into thin air, he no longer needed to storm out of the room, the lovemaking over, crushed by shame and ridding himself of every trace of Geraldine in a tearing haste, nor did he need to sit on the bed for an eternity, puffing away at his cigarette in silent fury. Instead he now liked to talk with me, still warm with love.

'Lovemaking is such a deep personal commitment that to leave you like this each time – that's cruel!' he had said to me some months ago after first getting to know me better. Instead, the after-love hour now became for us a treasured hour. With me nestling snugly in bed and looking up at him sitting by my side, the soft music still playing on, I was privileged to gain an insight into a Gerald at his most relaxed and revealing.

'I used to feel guilty because I thought that I was using you,' he had said to me on one such occasion, 'I did not realise all the possibilities of our relationship, and what we have now is *fabulous* – would *you* have it any other way, Mona?' And I was delighted to hear that he felt the perfection of us as keenly as I did.

Or he allowed his imagination to roam freely, anticipating with relish the scenes we would live out together some way in the future, there being no limits to the many themes possible, now that we had merged into one another so utterly. The ultimate fantasy was the one of the white wedding, Geraldine and Mona joined together in holy wedlock as husband and wife. But that was something as yet only to be savoured in anticipation, the real thing being a long way off, not anything to be undertaken lightly!

There were other times when Gerald, full of good food and wine, would probe deeply into the characters of Geraldine and Dina: 'Geraldine is an absolutely fabulous safety valve. While I am Geraldine, Gerald is sleeping, he is taking a rest. I think it would do a lot of people a lot of good if they could switch off and become someone else for a while.

'When I was a closet transvestite Geraldine used to be tarty in order to give herself the perfect turn-on, but now that I am with you she has changed completely. The changes that have taken place in me over the last six months have been so profound, that I could fill a book with all the feelings and the elimination of guilt, purely as a result of the relationship that you and I have. The most exciting thing that has happened is the birth of Dina – and Dina dictates the way she wants to be, and the way she wants to be is not tarty. Dina has a personality all her own, and I am very happy and pleased indeed to indulge her. After all, Gerald enjoys having the best of everything – what makes Dina a second-class citizen?

'Gerald will look after Dina. The time has come when he has to let her do whatever *she* wants to do.'

I listened, enthralled, hardly daring to breathe, not wishing to interrupt these revelations.

'Dina has a lovely figure, no doubt about that! And it gives me tremendous pleasure to dress her properly. I hope that one day I shall be able to say, "I want to dress *myself* properly!" Dina is very dear to me, as indeed Gerald is to Dina. There is a benign, parasitical relationship there. There is no doubt that Dina dresses to please Gerald.'

And, 'Gerald loves Dina – he is absolutely fascinated by her. When I am Gerald I would like to have Dina by my side.'

With Gerald's different personalities all brought out into the open, with each one of them having their own, special relationship with me, it enabled him to heal completely. And as he began to heal, so his natural buoyancy, sparkle and joy of life began to return. He was endowed with a ferocious appetite for life, for love, for affection, and blessed with a contagious sense of humour. Indeed, once he began to heal a lot of our time together was simply spent laughing.

Laughter and my tendency to giggle whenever I felt happy had previously been another bone of contention: Gerald had been touchy on the subject, imagining himself to be an object of ridicule in his 'dressed' state, and for several months I had had to suppress any urges to giggle whenever they came over me, in case he would take it as a personal slight, feeling it directed at himself, or rather at herself as she invariably would be at the time. Now he was able to laugh at his own predicament.

Every now and then as I managed to hold my breath for a brief moment to reflect on my new life, I marvelled at my riches. What a lover! We lived on a constant high, in permanent rapture! Surely, I thought, I must be singled out from all other women? I simply could not believe that there was another Gerald in existence anywhere, certainly not on this earth of ours, nor among all those countless stars and galaxies out there in the entire universe? I was convinced that he was unique and that I was uniquely blessed through him.

A sensation of religious fervour came over me, the unbeliever, as if someone, somewhere, had pointed a finger towards me, saying: that woman has suffered much – lift her up and show her a glimpse of heaven.

And suddenly a wave of huge elation had come over me: such happiness! I had the most wonderful lover any woman could ever dream of, the most wonderful lover in the whole wide world!

For a few moments I was aware: I could not possibly, ever, be happier than I was right now, I was at the pinnacle of my happiness, and I savoured it, extracted every grain of this happiness, revelled in it . . .

Half an hour later the telephone rang. Gerald said: 'Nothing can ever destroy the bond between us, our friendship is so strong, never mind what comes between us; I am not irreplaceable, I am not unique . . .'

I laughed, 'Oh, but you are, my darling, you are! You are quite unique and so is our relationship, and nothing can ever replace it!'

He said, 'Mona, I may go to America . . .'

I recognised the pattern only too well. After happiness – pain! I spent the rest of the night pacing up and down, up and down, turmoil raging inside me – trapped.

Gerald had been offered the chance of an incredible job, quite out of the blue, a result of his excellent reputation in his particular field – I was almost totally excluded from this world of Gerald's, but I was not in the least surprised that people should seek him out. I knew he was immensely able, a professional to his fingertips, experienced, widely travelled, and with an extraordinary knowledge of people. And now that he had healed, he was bursting with ambition and drive.

Someone, somewhere, was going to benefit from this new Gerald, and they would never look back.

And what about us? Well, what about it? Had we not always known that one day it must come to this?

Nothing was happening for a while, and I relaxed, pushing uneasiness and fear right out of sight.

But time passes as it must, and the date for Gerald's first interview had been fixed. It was my job to drive him to the airport. Gerald sat next to me, slim, neat and elegant in his stripy navy-blue business suit, so damned attractive, every inch of him the efficient young executive, and yet – only last night! I tried to be philosophical about it all, taking my lover to the airport so that he might meet the people who would take him away from me.

At the airport I reached out to kiss him goodbye. 'No lipstick, please,' he smiled at me. So near and yet so far. Be strong, Monica and say goodbye nicely. I raised my finger to his lips and stroked them: 'Goodbye my darling, much success – I love you!' And he was gone, turning round just one more time, lifting a hand towards me.

Of course they wanted him.

They offered him plenty of scope: heaps of money, responsibilities, a chance to use his superb brain. Success, success, all the way. A long way indeed from the dole he was on only such a short while ago.

Gerald stood before me in the room freshly back from the interview, tense, strained, white-faced. Quickly I hurried to put a gin-and-tonic before him, then ran his bath, hot and scented. My heart ached as I looked down at him lying there, so pale; all my dormant maternal feelings erupted hotly inside me and were now let loose on him; I wrapped the mantle of my fierce maternal love around him tightly, so tightly, until he began to unwind and feel warm and beloved and deeply secure, safe as a baby in his mother's womb, my darling, my adored man-child!

Softly I touched his face, his hair, his neck, and watched with great and profound satisfaction as he responded slowly, all tension leaving him little by little, and colour and life were returning once more to his darling face.

But it was time I remembered my role!

While Gerald relaxed in his warm bath I scanned our wardrobe for something special for him to wear tonight. The tightest of corselettes was a must after all he had been through, and to go with it I chose one of his favourite dresses, dark red in colour and flimsy, its shape beautifully soft and flowing.

As Gerald emerged refreshed his eyes fell on the corselette and dress spread out there so temptingly on the bed before him. He was thrilled with my choice and lost no time to transform himself with my help, to surface an hour later as Geraldine, radiant.

With elegant movements of her long and shapely legs she headed for the kitchen, to cook for us one of her cordon bleu creations to be enjoyed over a long, lingering evening of music, romance and fantasy, and to be followed by our marvellous loving.

A couple more months to go before he had to leave – but Gerald was busy winding up his affairs, getting ready.

Our beautiful relationship, such a vibrant, living thing, was going to be cut short, abruptly, as with an axe.

I watched him with a trembling heart. How could I bear to let him go? I knew only too well how much he hated emotional scenes – throughout our affair I had always had to be the stronger one, never allowing him to sense my sadness or my despair.

Yet, oddly, the real pain remained in the background. There was still so much loving to be done before he would leave me. Somehow I could not be sad while he was still with me, he was my very lifeblood, my soul-mate, and deeply integrated into my flesh. Instinctively, as I had always done, I responded to his needs – and his needs were for laughter, for pleasure, for romance and fantasy, for complete immersion into his transvestism and for exquisite, lifegiving sex.

I dared not contemplate the future after Gerald. A succession of grey and lifeless years ahead – lonely wherever I shall go, the spectre of ageing without him. I pushed these terrible visions away and as far out of sight as they would go – time enough for the suffering and the pain, later . . .

Dina meanwhile had steadily grown in confidence; from her uncertain beginnings she had slowly developed into a capable young woman, able to look after herself and her affairs, fitting well into modern life. When Gerald's brother asked him to produce a company report before leaving, Gerald decided that Dina could do it just as well, if not better.

She dressed for the purpose in a business-like way; she put on my black flared skirt and a red blouse and tied a little coloured scarf round the throat, and now Dina was ready to start. She had brought her bulging briefcase with her and for the next two days or so sat by the dining table, writing – writing non-stop, hardly pausing for a moment. 'What concentration!' I thought admiringly as I tiptoed around the place, careful not to disrupt such an important activity. At long last, as the evening approached, there were signs that the job had come to an end. Dina sat back sipping her gin-and-tonic slowly and smoking a cigarette, checking over her writing, winding up her report. I did not like to ask too many questions, company reports being rather beyond me, but I was curious to know how she felt about it.

Dina sat back and puffed on her cigarette. 'Gerald could never have done it so well!' she exclaimed, leafing through the pages. 'The male executive has to be clever enough,' she said, obviously pleased with herself, 'but the female has to be super-efficient and much better than her male counterpart in order to get to the top. Female super-efficient execs are to be feared!'

Meanwhile we had been hibernating now for the best part of a year, had been blissfully snug and warm inside our hideout and I had guarded it jealously, making sure that no one would pass through that front door while inside Geraldine, Gerry or Dina were freely moving about.

Did my new paying guests upstairs suspect my close relationship with Gerald? If they did, I did not care; it was my life. In the mornings, while the rest of us sat chatting amiably enough over our breakfast, Gerald was enjoying a luxurious lie-in only inches away in my bedroom, not to surface, usually as Gerry, until everyone had safely departed for work. As for Geraldine, she needed my protection, and I never tired of devising ways and means of hiding her and keeping her out of sight. She was our secret. By keeping everyone else at a distance, I made sure we were left to ourselves.

True, there had been a few moments when a friend would call unannounced, hoping for a warm welcome and perhaps a cup of coffee. I had to have in readiness a number of excuses, such as needing to dash off to the dentist's and such like, feeling dishonest and awkward.

Or, if the caller would not be put off, we had to use our escape route, Geraldine letting herself out via the kitchen and into the garden, and from there through the French windows into the bedroom where she could either hide or change back to Gerald, depending on the visitor. It was a bit like playing cops and robbers, all very exciting as long as it did not happen too often; which it didn't, as I had studiously neglected everyone with the exception of Louisa. We were self-sufficient, we needed no one.

But now everything was changed. The future looked too horrid to contemplate, though life after Gerald would have to go on, somehow. I therefore decided that it was high time for me to renew contact with the outside world and to prove to everyone that I bore them no grievance. I would give a party while Gerald was still around, one last splash before the pain would grip me. I would open my house to show that I was still alive and kicking, and I would show off my lover to them. I could not wait to watch the reaction of all these nice and clever people to Gerald. Especially the women.

I was so besotted with Gerald, I had got the unshakeable conviction that no woman anywhere, young or old, could resist him should he put his mind to the business of wishing to seduce her: I knew, absolutely and without any shadow of a doubt, that sooner or later she had to yield to him. I had seen the effect he had on shop girls. They reacted as if a bombshell had exploded in their face and at first behaved as if they had been struck dumb, only slowly regaining their senses. If he tried on a jacket or a coat they could caress him to their heart's content while smoothing the garment over his chest and shoulders; otherwise they responded to him with their eyes which at first turned from dull to excited, and after the initial shock was over they became relaxed with him and familiar, with a tendency to tell him of their family history.

When I told Gerald of my plans he was enthusiastic, grasping at the chance to prepare the food for the evening, being a dab hand at it and visualizing a very happy Geraldine having a whale of a time in the kitchen. As for me, I am a slow plodder when it comes to food: I am all right with good, solid, wholesome dishes such as I had cooked for my family, but not for me the pastries, quiches, pizzas and sauces all prepared in a jiffy. Gerald, in the secure knowledge of his culinary skills, had left everything to the last minute.

Geraldine was just rolling up her dainty sleeves when the telephone rang – an emergency summons for Gerald – there was not a minute to waste. Geraldine quickly reverted back to Gerald and departed, leaving me behind in a panic, working myself into a frenzy and ending the evening near to a nervous breakdown.

The next day, just as the party was about to start, there was the sound of a key turning – it was Gerald, just back in time to open the door to the first guest. Somehow I had managed. The tables groaned with food, the drinks were waiting and Gerald, to top it all, was in excellent shape.

In fact he was in buoyant mood, splendid and at his most debonair with the ladies; he bewitched each one in turn and did me credit. My dear middle-class friends were instantly enchanted with this charmer, in particular the ladies, mistaking him for a handsome playboy, an image he projected quite deliberately and in which he was totally relaxed, especially as unbeknown to anyone but me he wore his corset and nylons underneath his grey flannels.

Everything went swimmingly. I was proud of Gerald. He stoked the log fire, poured the drinks and handed round the food. Even here, right in front of everybody, we moved around the room in complete harmony, never losing sight of one another, our movements blending to perfection, like two musical instruments playing in unison. The night was happy, voices bubbled, laughter filled the room, all my friends together. And yet there was this great sadness inside me – I knew that the hour would pass, that there was nothing permanent about it all, and that soon Gerald would be gone, that this beautiful night was so fleeting, that there would never be a repeat . . .

'That lady looks very fragile,' said Gerald, startling me out of my gloom and pointing to a tall, thin blonde with huge blue eyes. I looked at Sybil. 'And no wonder,' I said, 'since she is just recovering from a bout of pneumonia caught at Greenham Common.' At this Gerald jumped up as if stung. 'Greenham Common!' he exclaimed and now directed all his attention to the hapless Sybil, whose husband, a veteran of the Human Rights Movement, quickly rushed to her defence. I did not wish my fun evening to end in a heated political battle. 'Co-existence!' I cried out loud, at which, thank God, everyone buried their hatchets and retreated, back to their drinks and light conversation.

In the end our party turned out to be a great success. My friends, who had not seen me for so long, marvelled at my new look: much younger, much slimmer, more glamorous. It was all most beneficial for the ego.

The last one to leave was Margot, chic and cool with all the sophistication of a woman of the world, she had made an impression on Gerald. Margot is ultra-feminine. '*Au revoir, Madame, tres enchanté!*', Gerald called out to her as she was about to leave, and Margot grew in height by at least two inches.

Dawn was on the horizon when my playboy lover grabbed a bottle, a tape and a couple of glasses and we withdrew into the bedroom to continue the celebration in our own inimitable style.

And I had renewed contact with my old world. Or so I thought.

And what was going to happen now to 'our perfect love-nest'? We had our comfortable double-bed – is this where the dream was going to end? One of the things Gerald had promised to make for our mutual comfort and enjoyment was a beautiful dressing table, the shrine at which to pay homage to our appearances, at which to indulge and pamper ourselves. I myself had never possessed such an item of feminine luxury: in my spartan past a chest-of-drawers had always had to do, with a mirror propped on top, serving the purpose but decidedly lacking in appeal.

On mentioning it to Gerald he sprang into action at once.

Oh, the thrills of shopping with him! Wood and brasses, screws and wires, and we discovered a superb top to go over the drawers and a stylish lamp to crown the large mirror. The wonderful, the exhilarating fun of it all! If only ...! *'Don't* brood, Mona, leave be and exist just for the moment, hold hands with him, he is still yours!'

Once in the shop I kept myself in the back, watching him.

Gerald the macho man was impressive. Dressed in his most ancient pair of jeans and worn out old shoes, he was busy supervising the measuring and cutting of wood, completely authoritative and down to earth, earning the respect of even the hardiest handyman around. I noticed with amusement that even his walk was slightly bandy-legged in the clothes he wore now, much like that of a man used to horses and rough living.

Triumphantly we collected our haul and loaded up the car. Once back home Gerald just could not wait to get started, loving to create things with his intelligent hands, so broad and strong, so clever and capable, and so different from the hands of Geraldine, their nails thrice painted and looking exceedingly feminine. Before setting out on the job, however, there was a slight change of dress: Gerald became Gerry in my sleeveless white T-shirt over a padded bra, a pair of ladies' corduroy slacks over suspender belts and stockings, his white sling-back sandals. He was now ready for action.

Gerry got to work at double-speed, wasting no time, very quick about the job, very sure of what he was doing.

A day later and he had finished the base and fixed the lighting. As the dressing table progressed Gerry became more and more excited, barely allowing himself to stop even for a meal, working all out without a break, measuring, matching, cutting and hammering, filing and smoothing, joining.

By the following evening he had created for us an object of great attraction and elegance; like its creator the dressing table had got flair. It stood there, regal and impressive, the long top providing us with ample space for all our many jars, bottles and brushes, glitter and sprays, powders and cosmetics. A beautiful clear mirror went all the length of the wall behind, crowned by a stylish brass lamp giving out a good light, warm and clear.

We simply could not wait to fill the drawers with our many items of luxurious lingerie, with stockings, girdles and suspender belts, with jewellery and our many knick-knacks.

And now the time had come for Gerry to transform himself into Geraldine, using his new creation for the very first time.

The hour was late, well past midnight. I lay on the bed, listening to the soft music playing, watching. Gerry was in the process of becoming Geraldine. She sat on the white leather-topped stool in front of the mirror, wearing her long-line bra, corset and panties, all in black and with stockings and shoes matching. Choosing her make-up carefully she took all the time in the world to make herself attractive, every moment a homage to the new dressing table before her. I watched her, fascinated, smiling as I noticed her evident enjoyment, preening herself in the large mirror, turning this way and that. But wait – what was this? Geraldine began to stroke the dressing table, lovingly, sensuously, as one would stroke a living, breathing thing, each stroke a caress!

From my vantage point on the bed I was beginning to feel distinctly uneasy. I was waiting for Geraldine to come over to me, but she seemed to be emotionally involved with her dressing table, quite unable to tear herself away. As the night drew on it became very clear to me that this was no ordinary job satisfaction, not just the thrill of a painter looking at his finished painting or the sculptor at his creation. A strange feeling came over me: is it possible, is it really possible, that Geraldine was actually 'turned on' by this piece of furniture? Because I could think of no other way to interpret her actions.

Was Geraldine in the grip of yet another kind of fetishism? She sat sideways on the stool, one arm was tenderly stroking the top of the dressing table before her, caressing it as she extolled its beauty, 'It is lovely, absolutely superb, much too good to leave!' she said again and again as if to send me a warning across the room. I could almost feel the vibrations coming from her and over to the dressing table, the same vibrations which caused me to become more and more uneasy by the minute. There was a tension in our bedroom tonight, the air was heavy with it, Geraldine was getting herself ever deeper into a state of feverish rapture and delirium, establishing a strong and secret communication between herself and her dressing table.

I should be happy, I kept telling myself, Gerald has done this for us.

But I could only feel confused and lost. And still she sat there, only half turned towards me, unable to let go, unable to tear herself away and make the change-over. A piece of inanimate furniture to be preferred to me! Was I in the presence of one of Geraldine's most unpredictable moods yet? She behaved so strangely that even I, used to her ways as I was, felt utterly disorientated and disturbed, wondering if perhaps I was in a dream, needing to look around me and touch the familiar objects by my side to remind myself that I was in my own bedroom and not in cuckooland.

It must have been nearing three o'clock in the morning before Geraldine finally managed to take the couple of steps needed to reach me and slip into bed. 'Do you want to make love tonight?' she asked me, suddenly remembering me, and I did! I knew that once I felt her close, tasted her and smelled her, she would become my gorgeous lover or mistress once more, my adored darling.

We made the attempt, and as always of late I thought, 'How much longer?' But Geraldine did not have her heart in it tonight, all her excitement was now over there on the other side of the room and indeed, the dressing table looked absolutely splendid, grand and luxurious and feminine, bathed as it was in its own golden light.

In the morning, having attended to my paying guests, I took a cup of coffee in to Gerald. He sat up in bed, smiling.

'How does the dressing table strike you now?' I wanted to know.

Gerald gave a casual glance in the direction of the dressing table. 'Not bad, not bad!' said he, and turned his attention to the coffee.

Gerald had to be away for the next couple of days, and it was just as well. It gave me time to piece myself together, to reflect and try to digest what I had just experienced. I needed time to take walks in the park, time to watch the clouds chasing across the skies, to listen to the birds and the rustle of the leaves above me, I needed to see the golden flicker of the sun reflected on the waters of the river, I needed to feel the cool of the wind on my face. I needed calm, and I needed Louisa to talk to.

Gerald – such an enigma! If anything, my love for him had grown even stronger, if this was at all possible. What must it be like to be lumbered with such a nature? Unless he had an understanding mate – how desperately lonely must he not be? I felt that I could not even begin to imagine the void which must have been his all those years – and what about the future? Of course, he could always sublimate, try and forget, immerse himself in a thousand activities, a thousand relationships. With all my heart I could only pray that he would find true happiness ...

Meanwhile our friend Marilyn had teamed up with Steven, a bi-sexual transvestite. They were in love! We watched them at the Pembrook restaurant one night, and we were glad for them. Marilyn looked lovely in her elegant white dress while Steven was very male, in white shirt and tie, though his plentiful locks gave him the appearance of a young cherub. Marilyn had had a rough time of it. She had in the first exuberance of her newly won womanhood tried her luck with a true macho type, a South American sportsman bulging with muscle, who had been attracted to her by her milky white complexion and her blonde locks. When she had entered his den to sample the Chilean cuisine he had promised her, he had lost no time at all in trying to rape her. Not yet fully healed, Marilyn had nevertheless defended herself for dear life and managed to get away in the nick of time. Not a promising start exactly. But Steven knew what it was all about, no need for lengthy explanations, and so here they were, clicking their glasses over their Thai pancakes, looking deep into each other's eyes.

Gerald's imagination really knew no limits! He was full of fantasies. For today, for tomorrow, for the day after. His ultimate fantasy was the one of the white wedding, with Geraldine as the bride, all in white, in a dress made especially for the occasion to suit her discerning taste. 'Not all flouncy and frilly, but truly elegant,' said she. Myself the groom in trouser suit. Two friends to be invited to witness the ceremony (Marilyn and Larry? Our choice was not exactly great.) 'I shall only do it with you,' Geraldine said, 'I shan't do it with anyone else!' Needless to say, the bride will be a virgin.

By now I was feeling strong enough to contemplate anything – anything at all as long as it was with Gerald. What was more, I was looking forward to our fantasies, loving them. I had become addicted to his ways, and I wished for nothing different, nothing better.

He kept on fantasising about this our wedding, making me recite the wedding vows, to make sure it would be all right on the day – to my own great surprise I did remember them fairly accurately, 'I take thee, Geraldine, as my wedded wife, for richer, for poorer, in sickness and in health, to love and to cherish, until death us do part . . .'

My sweet, my darling Geraldine! It was not to be, we never did get married, our courtship having been cut short so suddenly, so brutally, so irrevocably. I think of it with the deepest regret – seeing I could not have Gerald, it would have been the only wedding ever to have any meaning for me!

A subtle change was slowly coming over Gerald, who was now visiting his future employers at regular intervals. On his return he did not always find it easy to switch over from complete maleness into the fantasy of Geraldine.

After such a visit I sometimes found myself in the company of a beautifully turned out Geraldine, ultra-feminine to her very fingertips, facing me over her glass of gin-and-tonic by the light of the candle. She explained to me in the voice and intonation of Gerald about the intricacies of world economics or of international business. I was most fascinated by these topics but they were untypical subjects for Geraldine to elaborate on. I was reminded of our friend from the Pembrook, that overdone female for her evening out, holding forth by the hour about her work on the oil rig. Throughout the night Geraldine's eyes, as always expressing her mood so precisely, remained alert and cold.

I am afraid that this was a situation which threw

me. Was I to relate to the Gerald within or to the Geraldine without? Was I to respond to Gerald making sober and intelligent conversation, or was I to mould myself to the role he had chosen for himself for tonight in order to relax from the burdens of his maleness?

The score was 50–50. If Gerald had the upper hand we continued on the path of sober conversation. I learned a great deal, which pleased me, but at the end I felt like saying, 'Good night, Gerald, thank you for an interesting evening – see you again, soon!' He must have felt the same. Geraldine's finery came off in the bedroom, Gerald said 'Good night, Mona,' hopped into bed, turned his back towards me and – hey-presto, escaped into his world of slumber. It was not quite as simple for me: I continued to lie awake for ages, pondering over the strange nature of my lover, the endless changes, the many challenges and surprises.

If, on the other hand, it was Geraldine who triumphed, the evening took on a different course altogether. Anything, but anything at all, could happen. The relief of shedding a burdened Gerald was simply enormous, and an exuberant Geraldine emerged, eager to abandon herself completely to a night of fantasy, allowing her soaring imagination a free rein, enmeshing me, her willing and adoring target, in her web of romance and pleasure, of ecstasy.

The time for Gerald's departure was approaching. He

suggested that we invited Louisa over to meet him as Dina, so that she and I would be able to share this mutual experience after he had gone. After all, it was Louisa who throughout all these past months had had to be my safety valve, putting up with my changing moods ranging from happy delirium to deepest despair.

Louisa was somewhat hesitant at first, although agreeable in principle. Indeed, for many months past she had successfully managed to avoid confronting Geraldine or Dina, although she had met Gerald a good many times. There was still an emotional hurdle to overcome, she was attracted to Gerald and fascinated by him in the same way that all women were. She was afraid of seeing him so utterly changed, perhaps unrecognisable, maybe frightening, perhaps ridiculous. But she was also my good friend and in order to please me she agreed to come on the appointed evening.

Dina had put on her new blue summer frock, pretty but simple, she had refrained from using her purple nail varnish, her make-up was moderate, and she kept her personality in low key. She did not wish to frighten or shock Louisa whom she liked and respected. Although we had not spoken about it, I suspected that this was also an added test of Dina's ability to pass convincingly as a female, and to be take seriously in that role.

The evening arrived and we had set the scene and laid the table, the candles were burning, the music played softly and the wine was waiting to be poured. Dina had spent the afternoon creating for us one of her fabulous cordon bleu meals, the enticing vapours of which were now filling the kitchen and dining room.

Louisa arrived punctually, a bunch of flowers in her hand. She smiled as I opened the door for her, but I could see the apprehension beneath that smile. Louisa's own background was middle-class but by no means stuffy, affairs of the heart and even divorce were certainly part of it, and she was as broadminded and tolerant as the next person, but what she was going to come across here tonight was something so completely outside her own experience that the very thought of it made her mind boggle.

Louisa and Dina met, looked at one another, smiled at each other. I could almost feel Louisa heave a sigh of relief: it was not as terrible as she had feared, she had managed to face *her*, and now Dina proceeded at once to put Louisa at ease by talking to her about Gerald. The movements were feminine, the voice and words were Gerald's. He must have planned this carefully, I thought to myself, full of admiration. I had been so sure that Dina would turn into Geraldine in the course of the evening, and that Geraldine, as was her way when in the company of people sympathetic towards her, would become more and more excited trespassing all the borders of normal conventionality, and involve us in the caprices and passions of her own unique brand. But tonight we had gentle Dina with us, and she was handling the situation carefully and wisely.

And now Dina told Louisa of Gerald's plans for the future, and that it had not been easy for him to make the decision to go overseas: 'I am leaving behind my childhood friends, my family, my roots. And I am leaving behind my mistress who is also my lover, friend, and mother . . .'

For some minutes I left them alone, guessing that Dina would like to have a few words with Louisa in private. The photograph I took of them both on my return showed them sitting side by side in a relaxed mood, smiling.

Louisa departed fairly early, back to the safe bosom of her family. Dina went to change. Not her dress, but her underwear. As her blue frock was rather see-through I noticed at a glance that she had chosen the red Janet Reger outfit. This meant that she was in an adventurous mood, the modest Dina reserved for Louisa's visit had taken a retreat and the flamboyant and sexy Geraldine took over, having restrained herself quite long enough.

'I have introduced you to the pleasures of the flesh,' said Gerald to me one night after our hour of love, 'and now I am taking them away again.'

As he was talking to me he stood by my bedside looking down at me, still adorned as Gerry, wearing the colourful bird of paradise negligée with the many-tiered sleeves, long necklace and earrings dangling, his expressive dark eyes still full of the love we had shared only moments ago.

With a chuckle I remembered all the occasions when Gerald at the beginnings of our romance used to lecture me on my shortcomings, rebuking me for my inadequacies in an effort to shape me into his perfect mate.

And I remembered too, and all too clearly, our first fumbling efforts. Gerald as a lover had never been relaxed, being first tense, then briefly sweet, then hostile. As for me, I had been inhibited throughout. Now all that was so changed – we had become the most supreme lovers in the whole world! We were tuned one into the other by every hushed sigh, every flicker of the eyes, every unspoken word – we just knew.

My sweet, my wonderful darling – how I loved him for being concerned about me, for anticipating my loss.

At about this time I had a vivid dream about Gerald:

Gerald is a baby just beginning to toddle, complete with nappies. He tries to climb up a ladder, but a ladder without a top, blocked half-way up. I take Gerald down, afraid that he will get hurt and bleed.

The dream over, how much could I shield him in real life? Soon he would venture out into the world, and he might indeed get hurt, and bleed. In my sleepless nights I tried to visualise Gerald far away, alone.

Alone?

Of course there would have to be women for him. The pain of it all numbed me, for my sake and for his. For we both knew that after our initial painful start we had now achieved the unachievable – the ultimate. We had achieved a relationship so extraordinary, so special as to make it unique. Uniquely beautiful. We were both humbly and deeply aware of it.

It seemed after all, that I need not have worried myself too much about Gerald venturing out into the big world without me! With incredulity I watched a new Gerald grow.

While bringing Geraldine ever closer to me, tying her to me with a thousand bonds, I had all along also nourished Gerald, giving him, guiltless, all the strength he needed to break loose, to strive in the opposite direction and away from me.

I could only catch the occasional glimpse of this new Gerald, he did not belong to my world, to our world, he belonged to the world out there, to his work, to his future; there were traces of him left when he returned from one of his repeated interviews in Europe, and every now and then he was there with me in the room, on the telephone, making one of his many business calls.

With amazement I watched a much harder, more ruthless Gerald deal with the world. Steadily but surely, more masculine than ever before, a complete macho man now, he was forging ahead, relentless.

I named this new Gerald 'SuperGerald'.

SuperGerald frightened me!

Had he always been there, hiding? Or had he grown side by side with Dina the soft and gentle, like a Siamese twin?

Like a hurricane SuperGerald swept away everything before him, ruthlessly and with a ferocious force, clearing the way for himself.

If SuperGerald was hard and relentless, frightening in his energy, determination and dynamic force, unstoppable, then so in direct contrast to this extreme, Geraldine his female counterpart was the ultimate in softness and femininity, pleasure-seeking, erotic and self-indulgent.

If I had to choose between SuperGerald and Geraldine, it's Geraldine every time. All Gerald's sense of fun, his lust for life, his colourful, riotous imagination, all his sensitivity, his eroticism and sensuality – all these he could only fully express when dressed to suit his mood of the moment – yes, give me Geraldine any time!

Evening – and I was expecting Gerald for the last time – I felt numbed and yet, strangely, I did not feel too sad. Rather parting like this, honourably as it were, than him leaving me for a younger woman and being within reach. Somehow, Gerald had always been unreal to me, a fantasy, not quite of this world, and so his parting also was not of this world. Or so I tried to tell myself. The thought of him loving a younger woman at some time in the future was something that I had had to live with ever since we first embarked on our unusual relationship.

With his arrival, as always, a feeling of perfect harmony and calm came over me, the completeness of being with the one human being who constituted my 'other half', there simply was no room for pain while he was with me. All that could wait till later. For the last time I laid out his clothes, to watch the transformation from Gerald to Geraldine, the dressing from the skin out starting with girdle, padded bra and stockings, the careful make-up, clown's paste covering up any traces of beard, the eyes gloriously emphasized with dark shading, now illuminating the handsome face of Gerry. Gerry, my great lover, my soul-mate, my Bird of Paradise. Lipstick was carefully applied, outlined at first, then two colours superimposed to get the right effect.

The moment had arrived to become Geraldine once more. The shoulder-length wig was carefully smoothed over the lovely strong hair, the last tug and pull, the momentary tightening of the lips – Geraldine was here, complete, the perfect woman.

And confident, with a little smile, she proceeded into the kitchen, there to cook our evening meal, to be consumed once more by music and candlelight. 'I shall never forget,' said Geraldine.

For the last time we talked and laughed together over food and wine, our minds merging so easily, so easily, blending as harmoniously as did our bodies.

And, as so often before, Geraldine divested herself of dress and petticoat and changed into sexy underwear for our loving, thus generously allowing me as much freedom of her perfect body as possible, dressed only in bra and bikini briefs, suspender belts and stockings, a concession she had developed with our strengthening relationship, with the growth of mutual trust, a very long way indeed from her original complete cover-up.

The next morning was our last. Gerald's suitcase was waiting to be packed – how empty my wardrobe would be! With a heavy heart I watched as he lifted dress after dress from our mutual wardrobe and folded it neatly into his case. The new dressing table yielded its silken lingerie – each garment laden with memories of fantasy, of rapture.

It was Gerry for our last loving – no wig – the red Janet Reger outfit I gave him for Christmas. Our music had to be James Galway, we both opted for it instinctively: it was the music of our beginnings.

And the miracle happened: here, only hours before saying goodbye we entered a new heaven, crossed new thresholds, Gerry the she-male and I – who am I? Unplanned, grown quite naturally out of our twin souls and chemistry, we embarked on a new beginning.

As I finally managed to weep he kissed away all my tears.

IX

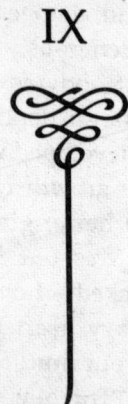

For three weeks I felt nothing. I moved about as in a coma, a soft warm haze enveloping my whole person. With ease I dealt with my daily tasks, my feet walking on cotton wool.

Then one Sunday morning, exactly three weeks to the minute after we had said goodbye to one another, a sudden cruel blow hit me in the stomach. Grief, the merciless, brutal grief which had lain in wait all along, had come to claim me after all.

There came that terrible moment one evening when I turned my head towards the kitchen, half expecting to see Geraldine busying herself with our meal, and saw not Geraldine but Arthur, that pigheaded intruder from upstairs waiting to be entertained by me, making himself yet another cup of tea. The pain, oh, the pain!

On the coffee table in my living room lay the latest bulletin of the Beaumont Society, arrived at last that morning, showing Geraldine's new membership number. Too late – too late.

The silence in the house was deafening. It screamed at me. I put on one of Gerald's favourite tapes which he had left behind for my comfort and solace, and turned it on – loud, as loud as I dared, to drown that silence. The sound was earsplitting, but still the silence inside me remained untouched. Once in a while, just for a few seconds, I managed to escape and recreate the magic: I poured myself a glass of sherry and sprinkled myself with our scent, I listened to our favourite music, I conjured up the image of Geraldine in my inner eye and for just one brief moment a great happiness would well up inside me.

During the day, unable to bear the emptiness around me, I dragged myself outdoors, to mix with the multitude of busy shoppers and the people going about their business in the High Street, to hear the noise of traffic, to look at shop windows. I went into our large store and straight up to the lingerie department, to gaze and to touch, to feel Geraldine near me. Every now and then the back of a man's head or a face in a passing car startled me – it is he! Only to realise a few moments later that I had been dreaming again. Once or twice a week I met Louisa, thankful to talk to her about Gerald. Occasionally I saw my children and waited for the moment when I could mention Gerald, careful not to appear too ridiculous, but needing to hear the sound of his name, perhaps a response. It was early May, fifteen months exactly since Gerald had first entered my house. One day passed like the other, nothing varied the pattern of my life. For days on end I spoke to no one. No one called. I had cultivated a life without callers.

Loneliness invaded my waking days as it invaded my nights, those nights when I saw him make love to some smooth-skinned young beauty, alluring and seductive as I could never be, never had been. In my nightly agonies I suffered all the tortures of hell, allowing Gerald first one, then two, then three weeks to get over us sufficiently to make the breakthrough. Women he would have to have. Women would pursue him as they had always done. All he needed to do was to reach out and take his pick. Night after night after night I saw him with some other woman, watched every gesture, heard every word. Night after night, feeling sick and desolate. His eyes, his mouth, his voice, his sex!

Often I got out of bed in the middle of the night when the agonies became unbearable, to fetch one of our albums, to look at our photographs, such wonderful pictures of Geraldine, of Gerry, of Dina. As for Gerald, he hated to be photographed, but Geraldine had posed on instinct, like an accomplished model. The pictures could not diminish the pain and the longing, they were only pieces of paper after all, they did not breathe, they were good images, but dead.

The tapes we had made together were a little better. Gerald's voice spoke to me, so warm, so full of love, so intelligent, so bursting with his humour. I could hear us laugh together; I could hear myself asking questions of Geraldine, and her answers to me, and sometimes she got carried away and talked about herself, endlessly.

But the voices came to an end and I found myself sitting up in bed, crying. Loneliness took over once more until I began to dream of death. Death the end to my loneliness.

At the same time I knew beyond any shadow of doubt that what had happened between us was so profound, went so deep as to make things difficult for Gerald; he would not find it easy to find a replacement for me. On the other hand I knew him to be a very rational man, strong-willed and persistent and he would forge ahead towards his goal. Life demanded of him that he tear me from his heart and find another.

I could not see my way ahead at all. If I had been cheerful and confident before Gerald had entered my life, now I became desolate. I could not cross my room from one side to the other without thinking of him. Richer by our incredible experiences and a great deal wiser, a new and completely changed woman, but the loneliness and frustration eating into me like a cancer, deadly.

As I moved about the empty rooms I felt myself to be incomplete, stunted. I compared our love to the wisteria which Gerald had planted at the back of the house, on the veranda close to the wall, and which had rapidly struggled upwards, rampant and prolific, until it had reached the roof. Twice I had to have it trimmed down to stop it from growing further, out of reach, higher and higher still. Our love had been like that: growing out of control and ever stronger, beautiful but quite unmanageable and not at all compatible with any practical requirements. Now that Gerald had cut off our loving by leaving me I had cut down the wisteria too, leaving only a small stump. Like our love it had not fitted in with its surroundings.

Weekends were hellish and Sundays the worst of all. Some Sundays, after not having spoken to a soul for days, I would take myself out of the house just to see life, movement, hear noises. Quite often I would take a bus or a train and go to Knightsbridge and Sloane Square, to stare into the shop windows at Harrods and other exciting stores, to divert my mind, and sometimes during the week I would go back to Barkers of Kensington and retrace our steps, look up Larry even, while frequently consulting my watch as to the time, longing for it to pass so that I could swallow my pill and escape into sleep. These outings left me humiliated, a lonely pointless exercise, leading nowhere except to the passing of time.

Then one morning I took myself to the American Embassy in Grosvenor Square to apply for a visa to the USA, something which Geraldine had asked me to do. At least it was an activity connected with Gerald – who knew what might not come of it?

I took out my passport with a new photograph of myself – I could not bear to look at my own picture.

I had tried so very hard to manage a little smile, had taken one picture after another, five in all, but I could not eliminate from my face that look of great tragedy, and so there it was, staring back at me, the eyes huge with suppressed tears. Well, it would have to do.

In Grosvenor Square I looked up at the Embassy, in awe of so much solidity, so much grey stone. I felt crushed by all that stone and insignificant, tiny and powerless over my fate. It was hard to believe that in some strange way my lifeblood had now become linked with that faceless building representing America, that huge continent of which Gerald was now a part, a minute drop in its vast hive of activity, and no longer a vital part of my life, of the little house in Richmond.

Inside the building the lady behind the counter called out my name: 'Mrs Jay?' she smiled at me, 'your visa is ready!' How quick, how simple. If only now I had lots of money and knew his whereabouts, all I needed to do . . .

June. His first letter has arrived! Factual and without frills, it is written by Gerald. He lives in hotels, he hates hotels, he loathes them.

> *'It is early days yet to say how the job is going. I am still trying to find my feet . . . as usual a major part of the job is convincing people what I want them to do and getting them to do it. The managers are competent but uninspiring. None of them has the slightest spark*

of inventiveness or drive . . .

You should know that I have missed you very much and continue to do so. I take out the photographs occasionally, but that doesn't really help very much. The nights are often lonely and getting to work in the morning is frequently a major effort of will . . . the last three weeks have not been without their moments of anguish.'

For Gerald, not easily given to going into his feelings, that was quite an admission.

I could breathe again, I could hold up my head once more, look forward to our meeting in August.

At home I seated myself before a blank sheet of paper to write my first letter to Gerald. How to convey to him all the many thoughts and feelings which crowded my mind? I needed to tell him of my love, of the emptiness around me, of all the little things happening in my daily life, of the clothes I wore, of my hatred for Arthur who now so smugly occupied Gerald's chair at breakfast and his former little bedsit.

Suddenly the written word loomed large and became all-important, my only contact with Gerald. I, who had hardly written anything since my school days beyond the annual Christmas cards, found myself thinking how wonderful it would be if I could relive our extraordinary relationship on paper. I took a deep breath and wrote: 'How I wish I could be a truly great writer, able to immortalise my darling lover! Alas, I am not . . .'

I ended my letter, 'My darling Gerald, Geraldine, Gerry and Dina – I love all of you! Monica.'

The next letter from America arrived soon afterwards. As I opened it the first page practically jumped at me with its large, widely spaced wording written in Gerald's tall and elegant lettering:

Before you start on this letter, darling, please go and change, and dress the way I always enjoyed seeing you. And please wear something of mine, so that you might feel closer to me. James Galway wouldn't hurt either. So go to it!

This letter, although signed Gerald, was in fact written by Geraldine. I read on:

It is strange, I also felt wonderfully sated with you for some three weeks after we parted. Our lovemaking had ascended to yet another plateau of passion and affection. We had dedicated ourselves to finding out so much about each other's personality. I know that the real breakthrough was achieved and the loss of Mona is something that I find leaves a gap in my life that is unlikely to be filled.

You wrote some beautiful things in your letter, so I quickly changed and put on your lovely sleeveless cotton dress and here I am feeling as close to you as I can, with memories of you like a warm overcoat on my soul. From the hurt, bewildered look of our first attempts at lovemaking through to the awakening of hope, contentment and lasting desire for each other. Your removal of my guilt and fear, and your own gradual awareness of your body, the passion that you could arouse in me with it and thus the slow erosion of your own feelings of embarrassment. Do you remember

– we went from a pitch black bedroom to making love in daytime and at night with the lights on? Or slowly arousing each other in front of a warm log fire?

With what infinite understanding and patience you slowly taught me to open my heart and mind to you. And with what fear and trepidation did I embark upon the myriad layers of self-protection with which I had sheltered myself for the last twenty years. The loving understanding that you gave me made it such a fulfilling act in oh, so many ways. Can you understand when I say that you gave me so much and that I gave you so little in return? You are right when you say that you don't know which person you miss more – Gerald, Gerry or Geraldine. They are all parts of the same person.

But what about you? We have the strict Mrs Jay the landlady who is sharp and intolerant of fools, and then we have Monica the Jewish mother who has her feet firmly placed on the ground and obtains a tremendous satisfaction from looking after her loved ones and delights in their success but is still able to see their faults which only serves to increase her love and protection. And then we have Mona – who was always there really, she just never had the opportunity to develop – who is honest, passionate and every inch a truly wonderful woman, full of humour and warmth. I love all three of you. Each one satisfies a deep need inside me.

Pages and pages of love.

Heathrow Airport, August 1983, and we were in the middle of a heatwave. The plane was late. I stood a little way back from the exit where the passengers came into sight. I wanted to have a first look at Gerald before he could see me; he was to have been there half an hour ago. I wore my thin royal blue dress with the gold belt and a gold shoulder bag. I had managed to keep my figure. The tension inside me mounted to fever pitch, every time a new person came into sight my heart gave a leap as if it had gone mad. I could feel the colour leaving my face, I must have looked terrible. A tall, middle-aged man had noticed me and my state of tension and watched me with interest while pretending that he was unaware of me. As time went by I began to feel faint.

Hundreds of people poured out of the exit, but still no Gerald. The tall man had lost patience and had given up.

Suddenly, there he was — so bronzed, his hair cropped shorter than I remembered him, that I did not recognise him at once. He came towards me, his face alight, his arms around me. There had been a muddle in Paris where he had put his children on the plane, back to their mother. 'I'll give you a proper kiss in the car,' he said, and so he did.

He wooed me, he beamed at me, his eyes devoured me, he could not keep off me, his hands and mouth were all over me.

Back home Gerald seated himself in his old chair by the dining table, I put a gin-and-tonic before him. I could not trust my eyes, he looked at me as if he were seeing a vision, something from out of this world, something exquisite and to be worshipped. After all I had endured – could this be real?

I could not take it all in, this incredible truth that Gerald sat before me, adorable and adoring, an aura of success surrounding him like a halo. Something inside me kept itself aloof, warned me not to get too carried away. I had been through so much pain, I had been ill with longing. We had only three days and three nights. Then what?

Gerald looked up at me from his gin-and-tonic, gave me a disarming smile, and said, 'I must tell you, Mona, that I have not touched another woman!'

So there it was. The truth. Three months of agonising, sickening dreams, of seeing him . . . the truth being that we had bonded so deeply that neither of us will be able to escape the impact of the other, ever. Not ever. But if so, had I really done Gerald such a great and lasting service?

As the evening approached I gave Geraldine my new dress to wear – a birthday present from Gerald which had arrived a month ago, exactly on time, in the shape of dollar bills folded inside the lovely card, with instructions to treat myself to 'something fine, sexy and feminine, or alternatively something strong and dominant'. I had taken myself off to the West End to celebrate and had had a wonderful birthday, with Gerald looking over my shoulder. That day we were together, close. Together we chose the dress: Italian, colourful and very smart. I had come home and tried it on, preening myself in front of the mirror, with Gerald still by my side. I had gone to bed in happiness, but I had woken in the deep of night, flooded in tears, alone.

I had saved up my new dress, waiting for Geraldine to be the first one to wear it and I was glad: she was overwhelmed by my gesture. As for me, I wore the new lingerie which Gerald had brought me from the States: a pair of camiknickers in a delicate colour of unripe apricot, silken to the touch and light as air, rich with broderie anglaise.

The magic was back once more, nothing had changed, we lived on our cloud for three days and three incredible nights and even Gerald made love to me once – but on the morning of his departure Gerald became niggly, difficult, hostile. At the time I did not fully understand . . .

On the whole I was lucky for the remainder of 1983 and the following spring: Gerald came over several times, sometimes there was a gap of only three or four weeks, which was splendid, considering.

When Christmas 1983 came I had a new carpet for 'our' bedroom, the carpet which Geraldine had been dreaming of in the past, the pile so deep you felt you would sink into it forever, the colour a greyish blue, complementing to perfection the white of the dressing table with its golden brass knobs, that wonderful present from Gerald/ine. To the end of my days I shall not be able to enter my bedroom without seeing in it Gerald or Geraldine, belonging.

For Christmas he gave me what I had wanted from

him most of all: a ring. A sapphire flanked by two little diamonds, it went on the same finger which for so long in the past had borne the wedding ring, the symbol of my slavery. I treasure that ring beyond all else, it will never leave my finger while I can breathe.

But our relationship suffered. Starved of one another, yet with so little time together, trying to cram so much into such a short time, with the next parting always imminent, made us sometimes nervy and on edge. It was during one of Gerald's visits that we had our first big crisis.

I am sure that this could never have happened had we been allowed to remain together, or had we been married in the 'normal' way. As things stood I belonged to Geraldine only, and a Geraldine under stress at that.

It had been a generous Gerald who had promised me in his letter a night out 'to show Mona the lights of London', and I had thrilled to the prospect, my inward eye seeing me taken out by my dazzling escort, Gerald, in dinner jacket, smart and debonair, the most handsome man around while I, glowing with pride and the envy of everything female within sight, allowed myself to be spoiled just for once – oh just once – just a very little!

But this, alas, was not to be. It was Geraldine who took me to see the lights of London, and it was the Pembrook we drifted towards.

No sooner did we approach the dining room of the restaurant when an uneasy Geraldine demanded of me, 'You do the talking!' And so I did the talking, I hung up our coats, I opened the doors for Milady.

The Pembrook restaurant is a quiet, pleasant place to dine in and the outside public is attracted to it by its excellent cuisine and service. Marilyn was our waitress.

It never occurred to Geraldine that I, a true gender woman, was craving for exactly the treatment that she was craving too. The night ended in a fiasco with both of us tense, unable to communicate and utterly estranged, with Geraldine going to bed sulking, while I was devastated and spent the whole night, our last, on a chair in the next room, tormented.

Perhaps the best thing that could be said for our night out is that the utterly ordinary couple sitting at the table next to us remained quite oblivious of Geraldine's true identity.

In the morning I took Gerald to the airport where I left him en route to his new life. Both of us were shattered.

Back home I collided with Greg from room No. 1, who looked at me and gave a loud gasp. 'Go and sit down!' he ordered me and went and made me a cup of tea. I sank into the nearest chair, thankful beyond words for even this little attention, for him noticing.

The rest of the day I spent in bed, bedclothes over my head, wishing I could sleep forever.

And yet I could not be angry with Gerald. I knew, with all my love for him, that this crisis could only have come about because of his own deep unhappiness, his futile struggle with himself, his renewed efforts to suppress Geraldine. Sometimes I feared for his health.

In the meantime I had begun to write about us, scrapping most of what I wrote, tears streaming down my face, on and on like one possessed. I thought of Gerald all day long, non-stop, he was with me as I crossed the road, waited in the shops, drove the car, moved about my daily business, always, always, with only a few hours of drugged sleep to alleviate the pain. I had no immediate goal in sight, but the idea of perhaps getting 'it' out one day began to take shape. I had been through an extraordinary experience, I had something of importance to say, and so I wrote and wrote. The hardest times were those when I had waited for a letter, weeks and weeks often, and no sign of life from Gerald. Would I ever hear again? I always did, in time. I knew then that he had been fighting his alter-ego again, and that meant that he had been fighting me, Geraldine's accomplice, her lover, her confidante, that he had drowned himself in work exactly as I had always known he would. From time to time I stopped my writing altogether, feeling the task was too big, that I was not equipped to do it.

But someone had to say it all. I looked around for that someone, I joined the writers' class at my local college with the one purpose in mind of asking my teacher to write my story for me or to suggest someone who might. My teacher, a busy playwright, declined, and I never divulged to her the subject of my proposed book. Instead, she suggested that I advertise for a ghost writer. However, bit by bit, as I listened carefully to what she had to say, I thought that I might persevere and give it a try, myself.

And so it began. My book of sublimation.

X

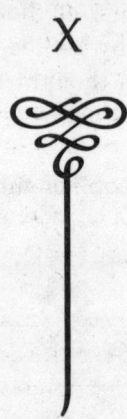

While I was keeping myself busy with my writing over here, Gerald was working his guts out on the other side of the Atlantic. You don't become Mr President for nothing. Mr President of the US side of a largish company dealing with the production and sales of electronics, all the latest, both in the US and in Europe.

Gerald was working all out, not sparing himself, giving it all he had got. His holidays were what he lived for: to be with his children, to become for a brief spell a normal warm Daddy to Emily and Tommy, to let himself spill over with his love for them, and to be adored by them in return.

But at work he had a lot of trouble. Some of the older people who had been in the company before him refused to cooperate with this bright young thing so newly imported from England, and they caused him all the headaches they could. For sure, they did not know Gerald, or they might have thought twice before opposing him. Gerald was constantly on the move, not allowed to grow roots in any one place, not seeing much of the pleasant one-bedroom apartment he had taken, situated on a luxurious estate, all mod cons, swimming, tennis, social club.

The ladies of the social club were after him like a shot. 'You would never believe to what length they will go, Mona!' he said, and I had laughed, understanding their motives perfectly: 'Oh yes, but I would, I would!' Gerald had looked uneasy telling me about it, and uncomfortable. What none of these ladies knew, what they could not possibly ever know, was that Gerald understood them only too well and, loving and venerating women the way he did, he felt embarrassed on their behalf.

On one memorable occasion the ladies of the Social Club had managed to lure Gerald to a meeting: thirteen women and two men! It was an unforgettable as well as an unrepeatable experience.

There came the day when Gerald, desperate for female company, summoned a call girl. She arrived: young, attractive, well made up, elegant, but he could not bring himself to have impersonal sex – not after *us*! He managed to ask her to scratch his back for him and sent her away, paying her $100. 'Any time!' she said, and left, delighted.

He had to solve a thousand problems, make a thousand decisions. He created a new company branch down South and he selected the site, designed the lay-out of the new building, chose the colour scheme. He loved the power and freedom it gave him in so many ways, he could hire and fire as he thought right. He was proud of his status and the trust and the responsibilities that went with it, but it in turn enslaved him and drained him and made him need Geraldine more than ever before.

But SuperGerald would not allow himself to acknowledge Geraldine, he fought her, he suppressed her, he denied her. He thought that if he worked himself to a standstill, played hard at tennis and went waterskiing whenever he had a few hours to himself, he could keep her at bay. He tired himself out mentally and physically, but Geraldine would out.

She would parade herself before him shamelessly and give him the come-hither look, the hussy! She would mock him and tease him, she would toss her curls and wriggle her hips and rustle her skirts endlessly, and lead him quite a dance, until he felt helpless with desire for her and weak with longing and would have to go towards her and merge himself with her.

On his next visit to me he was badly in need of our old submission scene, riddled with renewed self-hatred and guilt feelings, and I, seeing him torn, could understand his need – truly, truly I could, and I was inspired as never before, I gave of my all. But if an excited and sexy Gerald had entered my bedroom that morning, it was a guilt-ridden and hostile Gerald who emerged at the other end. Later on he confessed that he was hating himself for having degraded me!

He now called it 'The Executive Syndrome' – but it was Gerald who was the executive, not I, and as long as our charade served to enhance our love for one another as it had done in the past, well and good, I could go along with that and enjoy every bit of it, but if not, then it was not for me. *No!*

And of course in time there was another woman for Gerald, but she could only love half of him. Again he had chosen a woman whom he would not marry: clean, intelligent, once again too old to bear him children, she had a grown family of her own. Was he, perhaps, trying to recapture what he had lost with me? He did not live with her, he now had neighbours to consider, but took her to a hotel once or twice a week, time allowing. She served his basic needs for sex and some companionship and for frequent lifts to the airport, but his emotional involvement remained minimal. It had taken him five months to take the step.

Telling me about her Gerald's eyes had devoured me with love, 'No competition to you!' he had said, and seeing my look of resignation had added, 'All right, supposing we were to give it a rating: if you are ten, she is two – what you and I have, Mona, is a relationship in a million!' And I had to be content with that.

Even so, my heart reached out to him, I saw a Geraldine hiding in her own four walls, loneliness closing in on her, with our occasional and brief meetings her only escape into true happiness.

And in the summer of 1984 I finally made it to America. America, where I had never been. I made my way up North from Miami but saw precious little for hoardings, hoardings all along the endless highway. In Florida I travelled through time in Planet Earth, made my 'Journey into Imagination' in the Epcot Centre, I became a small child again in the Magic Kingdom.

I sat on a bench in the Magic Kingdom munching my Kingsize Burger and had my first good look at the Americans *en masse*, a colourful conglomeration of peoples, watched them parade past me, the old and the young, the blacks and the whites, the thin ones and the fat ones. Papa, Mama, children, their layers of fat rolling down their ankles so you could hardly see their feet.

I liked the youngsters, they seemed easy, liberated, no hangups. One thing struck me: this was the South, and I could see no colour bar, no condescension by whites towards blacks, they mingled freely, chatted and laughed together, apparently completely at ease with one another. If they could do that, I thought, they had achieved a lot.

We met up in Charleston, South Carolina, under a sun that was killing. Gerald was there, sitting on a bench, looking a little flushed and excited. Good! We took off on the endless road, and within minutes my darling had got himself a $30 speeding fine, and within moments after that very nearly another one. You can't confine someone like Gerald to a 50 mph on a highway!

We spent a whole week together in an anonymous

capsule by a swimming pool, somewhere in North Carolina. There was a change in Gerald, who had by now crystallised into two sharply defined personalities: there was SuperGerald and there was Geraldine. And Gerald – my beautiful darling Gerald, that lovely man who had shared his life with me for such an all too short time – had evaporated into thin air, with all his warmth, his charm and charisma gone, wiped clean off his personality as if off a slate.

Lording it over his empire, king of decisions, ruler of underlings, SuperGerald the hard and ruthless was winning the day – but at a cost. With astonishment I looked at him: tense and strained, putting all his energy into his work, making a superhuman effort to turn himself into a proper macho man with no time for fun or for growing roots, he had become hard and bitter, mercenary even, hiding behind possessions with a desperation born of insecurity, with all his laughter, all his joy drained out of him, a closet transvestite all over again.

Geraldine, thank God, had remained intact. Warm as ever, romantic and exotic, my lover, my mistress, her magic was unimpaired.

But the sudden changes of personality were dramatic and could be frightening, even to me: one moment it would be Geraldine whom I was holding in my arms, warm and sweet and loving, and the next moment, her loving done, it was SuperGerald whom I was holding, an eagle, hard and cruel, about to seek out his prey, impatient to take wing. . . .

Back home again I had plenty of time to reflect.

The days dragged by. I could not wait for dawn to appear after another night of anguish. Dawn, the herald of another day, dawn the herald of new hope, dawn the herald of the postman.

But the postman's steps would come and go, and no letter from Gerald.

When eight weeks – *eight* weeks! – had gone by without a sign of life from Gerald, the moment arrived when I decided to face the fact that the end had finally come, that I would never hear from him again.

I sat myself down, slowly, deliberately, my head buried in my hands, trying to come to terms with the cruel facts, with the emptiness looming ahead where Gerald had once been, where between us we had created our paradise on earth. And a great bitterness crept in where love had been: how *could* he cause me so much pain, such heartbreak? But at this point my mind could go no further. My reasoning had come to a halt.

While I was sitting mourning him thus, the telephone rang. Gerald was speaking to me, his voice small and lifeless. He felt unloved. Unloved! I could tell he was in the throes of one of his depressions. He missed me, he loved me, he was 'pretending to live with me', a sad and pathetic exercise in loneliness.

The vision of the ladder came back to me – the ladder without a top, its rungs blocked half-way up, and how I had rushed to save Gerald the baby from getting injured, from bleeding.

A great sadness took hold of me, leaving me grieving, so powerless now to help Gerald. Was he destroying himself in his quest for 'normality'? Had I been witness to the disintegration of a beautiful man?

It's Sunday again – another endless Sunday.

So much has changed for me, I cannot believe that only three years ago I had not known Gerald. I look in the mirror to find the changes there in the reflection of myself. Fine lines have appeared in my face over the past eighteen months, the pain has made its mark. I smile at my image, but the pain still shows. And yet, only eighteen months ago my face had worn other lines, the lines of a great happiness, and I had worn them proudly and openly for all to see, my lines of distinction, the mark imprinted upon me by Gerald.

I turn away from the mirror and go back to the living room to finish my letter to America. My story is done. I lift my pen and write, 'You know me – I die, and then I come back, stronger!'

So often I have a wonderful dream and I am back on our soft cloud, securely draped in Gerald's love, and I smile as I watch him change into Gerry, into Geraldine, into Dina, my beautiful Bird of Paradise, bedecked in jewels . . .

Also available from Mandarin Paperbacks

ERROL FLYNN

My Wicked Wicked Ways

'Errol Flynn's autobiography is eventful (of course), entertaining (naturally) and – surprisingly – very well written with the flair of a born raconteur disciplined by something like the skill of a born writer'
Times Literary Supplement

'A big, brash, fundamentally sad book. It sounds very much like the man himself'
PATRICK CAMPBELL, *Sunday Times*

'Daring, bold, amusing and just a little sad . . . A story admirably told with vigour and style'
Irish Times

'. . . eye-and-cork popping, shockingly candid autobiography that names names, calls spades spades, queens queens, and kings bums . . .'
New York Herald Tribune

'A shocker . . . Flynn uses strong language, and writes with as much colour as his life deserves . . . There is no doubt that he lived one of the fullest, most active lives of his period, and this is an extraordinarily readable, enjoyable, revealing view of it'
New York Post

STEPHEN REBELLO

Alfred Hitchcock and the Making of *Psycho*

'This time you're going too far,' warned one of Hitchcock's associates about *Psycho*, the film now indelibly stamped upon the American subconscious. Charted here from grisly conception to dramatic aftermath is the course of one of the true landmarks in the history of horror.

'Joyously entertaining'
GERALD KAUFMAN, *Sunday Telegraph*

'Rebello takes us right through the project, from the original murderer – Ed Gein of Wisconsin, who made Norman Bates look like David Attenborough – to Robert Bloch's overloaded novel, to Hitch's five scrupulous weeks of storybashing . . . A heartening account of a shockeroo being distilled into pure cinema'
Independent

'Rebello's book combines a gossipy retrospective with a serious work of criticism, presenting an articulate guide to Hitchcock's idiosyncratic approach to film-making and the collaborative efforts that underpinned it. The author has conducted interviews with all those involved in the making of *Psycho* – its casting, scripting, shooting, art design, lighting, editing, selling – in the course of which we inch closer to the bizarre, unpredictable quality of its director'
ANTHONY QUINN, *Sunday Times*

RUTH BRANDON

Being Divine

A Biography of Sarah Bernhardt

The most spellbinding actress of her age, Sarah Bernhardt was a goddess of her own making, a beauty, a genius, a legend – the first genuinely original world idol. In a career that spanned sixty years, her superhuman creativity compelled her to play to packed houses all over the world, and well into old age. Her beautiful voice, her extraordinary seductiveness – on stage and off – and her superhuman energy earned her the adulation of countless admirers, and the fulfilment of a completely free woman.

'A remarkable story . . . Clearly the attraction for Ruth Brandon, in this breathless book, is of a woman of extraordinary independence'
ANITA BROOKNER, *Observer*

'*Being Divine* celebrates the first true celebrity of stage and screen'
She

'Eminently readable . . . A must for anyone interested in theatre, and a treat for anyone besides'
Spectator

TOM BOWER

Maxwell the Outsider

Larger than life, larger than legend

Robert Maxwell continues to make news even after his sensational and mysterious death. This book, which Maxwell tried to ban, now asks – and answers – the unresolved questions which remain. Completely revised and updated, it reveals:

- the truth behind Maxwell's extraordinary links with the KGB, the Kremlin and Eastern Europe

- the notorious 'Mirrorgate' affair and the reality of Maxwell's close relationship with the Israeli power elite

- his history of shady dealings which shocked the City

- his fatal greed in the USA which devastated his life's ambition

- the conspiracy of public and private companies that intentionally concealed a staggering £3 billion of debts

- and the sensational truth behind Robert Maxwell's death

JEREMY WILSON

Lawrence of Arabia

Man of action, man of letters, archaeologist, guerrilla-leader, kingmaker, diplomat and national hero, T. E. Lawrence is one of the most extraordinary Englishmen of this century. His daring exploits in WW1 and the Arab Revolt made him a living legend – which speculative interpretations have since done little to dispel. This, the abridged edition of the definitive biography, demystifies its subject without in any way diminishing the man.

'An extraordinary story . . . Jeremy Wilson has cut away the accretions of myth and romance . . . and the story of T. E. Lawrence – this odd, obsessive, driven man who sought anonymity and against all his wishes was granted immortal fame – is far more interesting than that of the conventional hero swathed in Arab head gear'
PETER ACKROYD, *The Times*

'It is hard to believe that Wilson's study will ever be bettered'
Independent

'Indispensable for the future students of Lawrence'
Financial Times

'This biography will endure beside *Seven Pillars* as his monument, and any future book about T. E. Lawrence will be but a commentary on it'
New York Times Book Review

A Selected List of Non-Fiction Titles Available from Mandarin

While every effort is made to keep prices low, it is sometimes necessary to increase prices at short notice. Mandarin Paperbacks reserves the right to show new retail prices on covers which may differ from those previously advertised in the text or elsewhere.

The prices shown below were correct at the time of going to press.

☐	7493 0961 X	**Stick it up Your Punter**	Chippendale & Horrib	£4.99
☐	7493 0938 5	**The Courage to Heal**	Ellen Bass and Laura Davis	£7.99
☐	7493 0637 8	**The Hollywood Story**	Joel Finler	£9.99
☐	7493 1032 4	**How to Meet Interesting Men**	Gizelle Howard	£5.99
☐	7493 1172 X	**You'll Never Eat Lunch in This Town Again**	Julia Phillips	£5.99
☐	7493 0618 1	**Justiced Delayed**	David Cesarani	£5.99
☐	7493 1026 X	**Billion Dollar Battle**	Matthew Lynn	£5.99
☐	7493 0626 2	**Murder Squad**	Tim Tate	£4.99
☐	7493 1031 6	**Catholics & Sex**	Kate Saunders and Peter Stanford	£5.99
☐	7493 1328 5	**Among The Thugs**	Bill Buford	£4.99

All these books are available at your bookshop or newsagent, or can be ordered direct from the publisher. Just tick the titles you want and fill in the form below.

Mandarin Paperbacks, Cash Sales Department, PO Box 11, Falmouth, Cornwall TR10 9EN.

Please send cheque or postal order, no currency, for purchase price quoted and allow the following for postage and packing:

UK including BFPO   £1.00 for the first book, 50p for the second and 30p for each additional book ordered to a maximum charge of £3.00.

Overseas including Eire   £2 for the first book, £1.00 for the second and 50p for each additional book thereafter.

NAME (Block letters) ....

ADDRESS..

....

☐ I enclose my remittance for ....

☐ I wish to pay by Access/Visa Card Number

Expiry Date

A List of Film and TV Tie-In Titles Available from Mandarin

While every effort is made to keep prices low, it is sometimes necessary to increase prices at short notice. Mandarin Paperbacks reserves the right to show new retail prices on covers which may differ from those previously advertised in the text or elsewhere.

The prices shown below were correct at the time of going to press.

☐	7493 0942 3	**The Silence of the Lambs**	Thomas Harris	£4.99
☐	7493 1416 8	**Wayne's World**	Myers & Ruzan	£4.99
☐	7493 1345 5	**Batman Returns**	Craig Shaw Gardner	£3.99
☐	7493 3601 3	**Rush**	Kim Wozencraft	£3.99
☐	7493 9801 9	**The Commitments**	Roddy Doyle	£4.99
☐	7493 1334 X	**Northern Exposure**	Ellis Weiner	£3.99
☐	7493 0626 2	**Murder Squad**	Tate & Wyre	£4.99
☐	7493 0277 1	**The Bill (Volume 1)**	John Burke	£3.50
☐	7493 0278 X	**The Bill (Volume 2)**	John Burke	£3.50
☐	7493 0002 7	**The Bill (Volume 3)**	John Burke	£3.50
☐	7493 0374 3	**The Bill (Volume 4)**	John Burke	£2.99
☐	7493 0842 7	**The Bill (Volume 5)**	John Burke	£3.50
☐	7493 1178 9	**The Bill (Volume 6)**	John Burke	£3.50

All these books are available at your bookshop or newsagent, or can be ordered direct from the publisher. Just tick the titles you want and fill in the form below.

Mandarin Paperbacks, Cash Sales Department, PO Box 11, Falmouth, Cornwall TR10 9EN.

Please send cheque or postal order, no currency, for purchase price quoted and allow the following for postage and packing:

UK including BFPO   £1.00 for the first book, 50p for the second and 30p for each additional book ordered to a maximum charge of £3.00.

Overseas including Eire   £2 for the first book, £1.00 for the second and 50p for each additional book thereafter.

NAME (Block letters) ....

ADDRESS ....

....

☐ I enclose my remittance for ....

☐ I wish to pay by Access/Visa Card Number

Expiry Date